Obesity Public Enemy #1 or Death

Obesity Public Enemy #1 or Death

Oscar Zaldaña Paredes
& Jose Paredes

Library of Congress Control Number:		2011908441
ISBN:	Hardcover	978-1-4628-7695-2
	Softcover	978-1-4628-7694-5
	Ebook	978-1-4628-7696-9

This book was printed in the United States of America.

To order additional copies of this book, contact:
Xlibris Corporation
1-888-795-4274
www.Xlibris.com
Orders@Xlibris.com
87441

CONTENTS

INTRODUCTION

Obesity has become the number 1 enemy of humanity, creating an epidemic that has taken an accelerated pace in recent years, affecting health, labor, development of civilization. Since the beginning of our history, being overweight was a part of a culture that determined status and power until today because it is killing humanity.

Our metabolism has changed, from the moment of conception to developing multiple problems and clinical conditions including lack of employment, social, psychological, and physical problems directly affecting the world's quality of life.

We now know that obesity (public enemy number 1 cause of death) has appeared due to our own behavior, bad eating habits, and lack of exercise.

If this trend continues, we will have a collapse in infrastructure, making it impossible to ensure the health of millions with diseases like diabetes, hypertension, stroke, heart attack, new cases of cancer, and other related illnesses affecting the entire human race.

The worst epidemic in the history of the world affecting the entire human race is killing us all.

CHAPTER 1

Definition

1) Obesity is simply defined as a condition of excessive fat accumulation in fat tissues of the body leading to health problems.

2) The underlying reason for obesity is an excess of calories ingested versus calories burned.

3) The BMI (body mass index) is used as a tool to determine if the weight of a person is healthy.

4) Body mass index is a relationship between the weight of a person and the height.

5) The classifications of weight are the following:

    <18.5 body mass index: underweight
    18.5-25: healthy weight
    25-30: overweight
    >30 obese

6) To get your BMI, you divide your weight in kilograms by the square of your height in meters (kgm^2).

7) For example, a person that weighs 69 kilograms and has a height of 1.60 meters will have a BMI of 26.

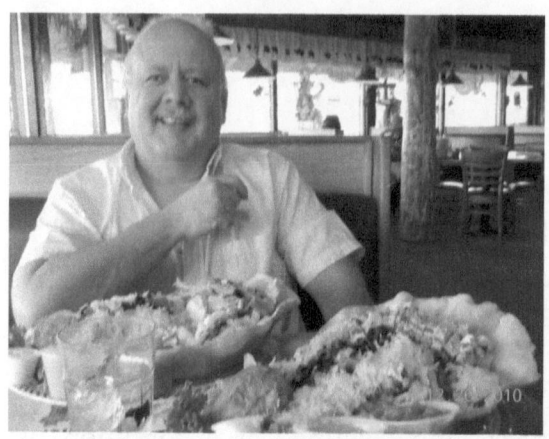

The Author showing the size of "NORMAL" portions

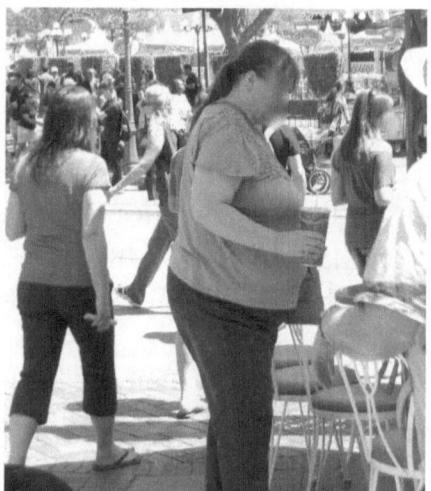

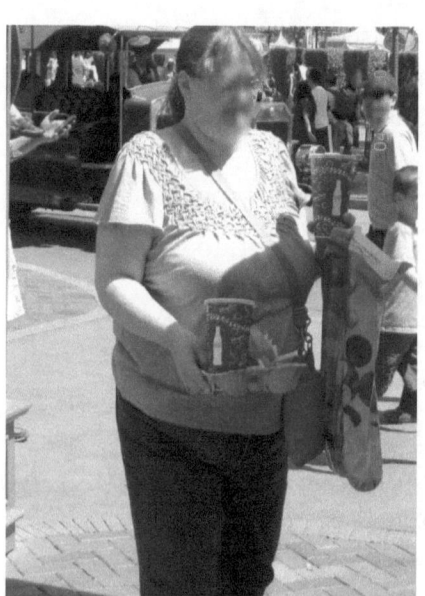

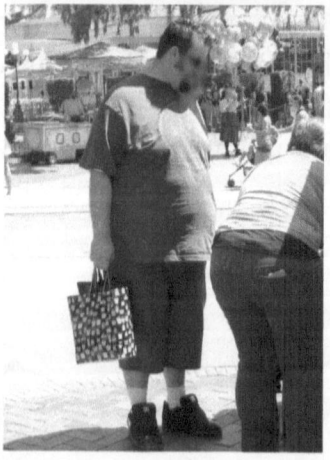

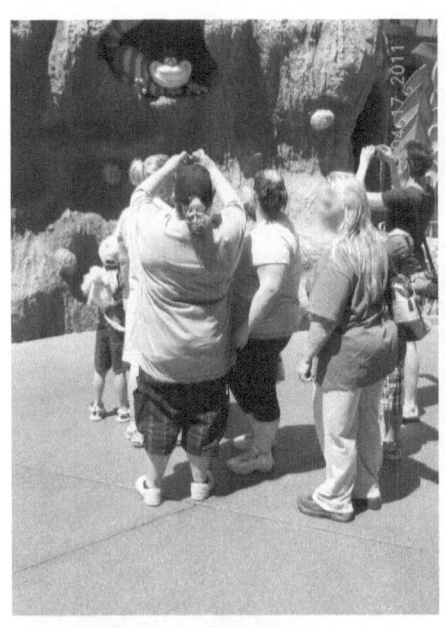
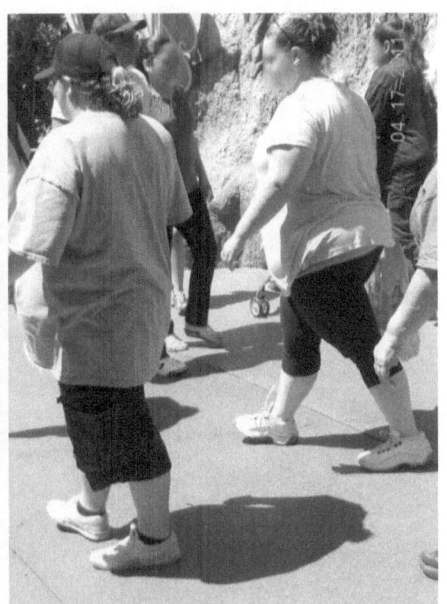
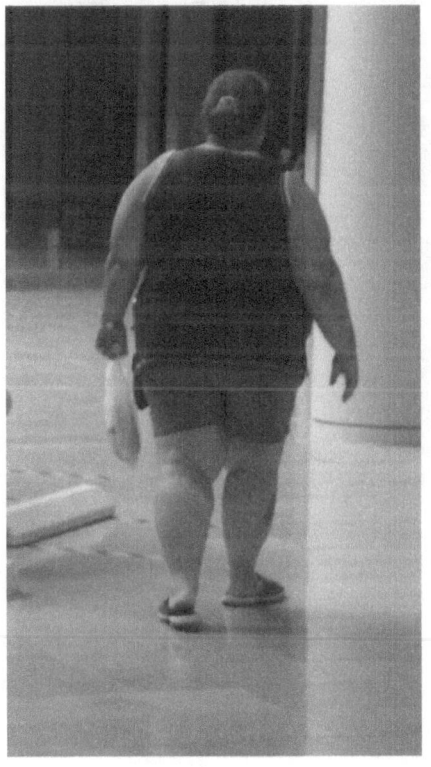
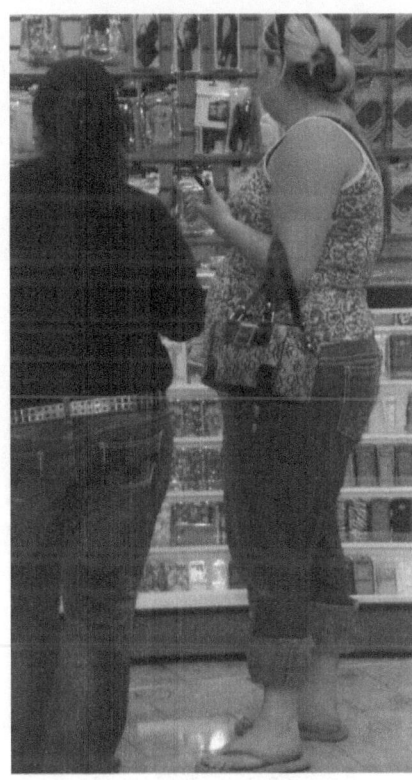

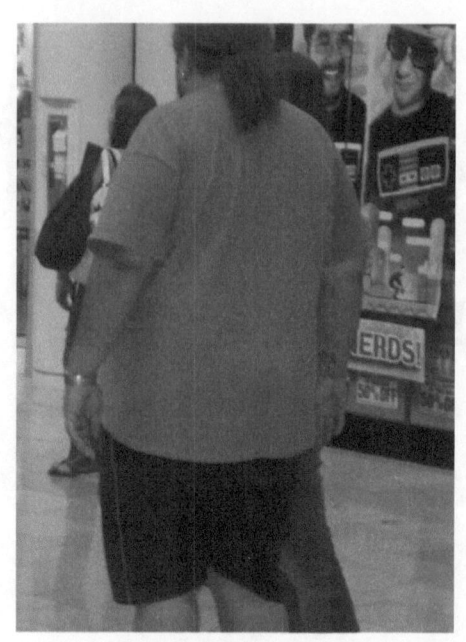

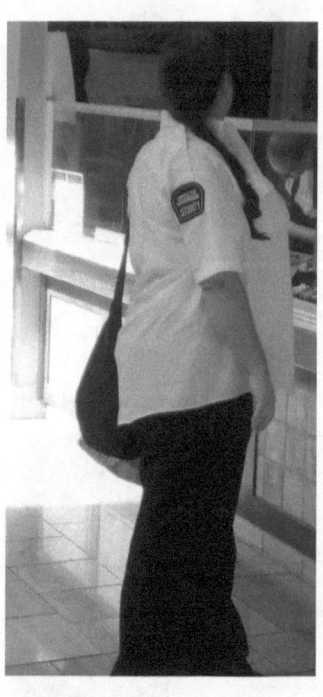

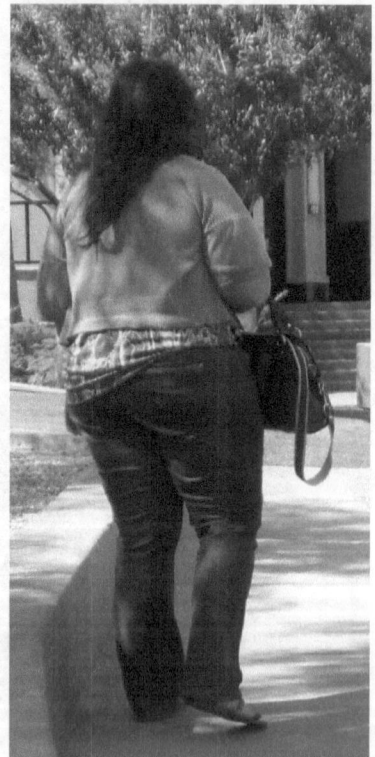

CHAPTER 2

History

8)   Obesity history can be traced back thirty thousand years ago to our prehistoric ancestors.

9)   About thirty thousand years ago, prehistoric statuettes, including the famous *Venus of Willendorf*, depicted anatomically accurate abdominally obese women (the oldest sculpture known to mankind). The function of these figures is not completely clear. They may have been fertility symbols, the figures small enough to fit in the palm of the hand—these have to be the predecessors of *Playboy* magazine!

10) Moses is considered to be the original writer on diet, recommending the Jews "bread, wine, milk, honey; quadrupeds that divide the hoof, and chew the cud; all the feathered kind, a few only excepted; and fishes that have fins and scales" (accurate text from the Bible).

11) Acceptance of obesity as a medical phenomenon has been slow. For thousands of years, overweight and obesity were exceptional, rarely seen and never studied.

12) In some cultures, indeed, obesity was prized, indicating status and wealth. Only the richest had the means to become obese, and a big belly advertised wealth more effectively than the richest clothing or the best jewels at the time.

13) The ancient Greeks were the first to realize the dangers of obesity and its association with disease. Hippocrates wrote about different diseases caused by a poor diet and how to improve health through changes in eating habits.

14) For the ancient Egyptians, diet was a mean to preserve health, recognizing that quantity, as well of quality of food, was very important. Fasting was a method to control quantity of food; they were explained by Diodorus Siculus to "prevent distempers by glisters, purging, vomiting, or fasting every second, third, or fourth day." Herodotus happened to agree that "Egyptians would vomit and purge themselves two or three times every month with a view to preserve their health, which, in their opinion, is chiefly injured by excess of food."

15) Pythagoras recommended a different way to preserve health through diet. No man, who values his health, ought to trespass on the bounds of moderation, either in labor, diet, or concubinage, especially diet.

16) Hippocrates defined correctly the equation of energy balance: "It is very injurious to health to take in more food than the constitution will bear, when at the same time one uses no exercise to carry off the excess."

17) Galen, a great physician, wrote about one of the earliest case studies of obesity management.

18) "I reduced a huge fat fellow to a moderate size in a short time, by making him run every morning until he fell into a profuse sweat; I then had him rubbed hard, and put into a warm bath; after which I ordered him a small breakfast, and sent him to the warm bath a second time. Some hours after, I permitted him to eat freely of food, which afforded but little nourishment; and lastly, set him to some work which he was accustomed to for the remaining part of the day."

19) Plutarch also studied the relationship between weight and health: "Thin people are generally the most healthy; we should not therefore indulge our appetites with delicacies or high living, for fear of growing corpulent."

20) Later, Thomas Cogan recounted Hippocrates and Galen adding his own observations, for example on exercise: "Flowing water does not corrupt, but that which standeth still; even so animal bodies exercised, are for the greater part healthful; and such as be idle are subject to sickness."

21) Henry VIII's physician, Dr. Andrew Boorde, wrote *Breviary of Health* in 1547, blaming alcohol as the cause of obesity: "All sweet wines and grass wines doth make a man fat."

22) John Armstrong wrote *The Art of Preserving Health* in 1744: "Unless with exercise and manly toil you brace your nerves, and spur the lagging blood. The fattening clime let all the sons of ease Avoid; if indolence would wish to live."

23) The English physician Tobias Venner was the first physician to use the word "obesity" in a medical context in 1660.

24) In 1765, Joannes Baptista Morgagni recognized not only that obesity was linked to disease but also by anatomical dissection that position of the fat was crucial. Abdominal kind is the worst kind.

25) William Banting wrote the first commercially available diet program.

26) In 1795, the link between weight and women's health became more important and more recognized because at that time they figured out that was a cause of death.

27) In 1811, Robert Thomas was the first to discover and describe the relationship between obesity and endometrial cancer (uterus cancer).

28) In 1811, Robert Thomas described angina (chest pain) the beginning of a heart attack and the relationship with obesity.

29) Gluttony was ranked by medieval Christian thinkers as one of the seven deadly sins.

30) Through the eighteenth century, there were many doctoral theses that studied obesity. The Dutch physician Malcolm Fleming described obese people as "unlucky inheritors of a predisposition, which was not completely within their powers to control" that is why it is so hard for people to control it.

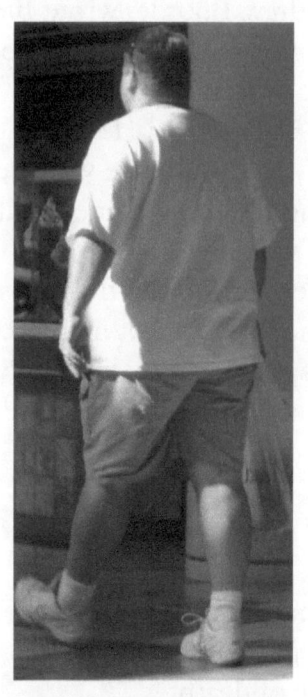
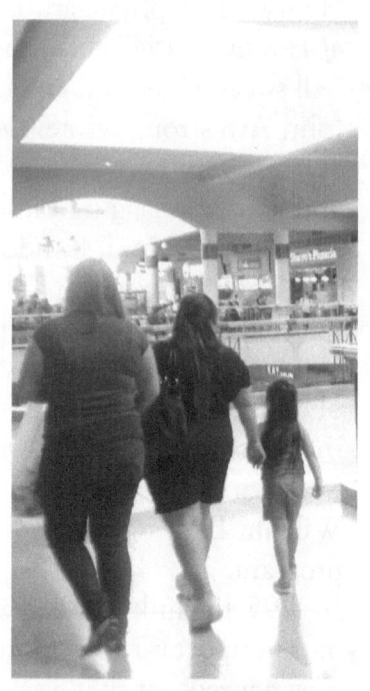
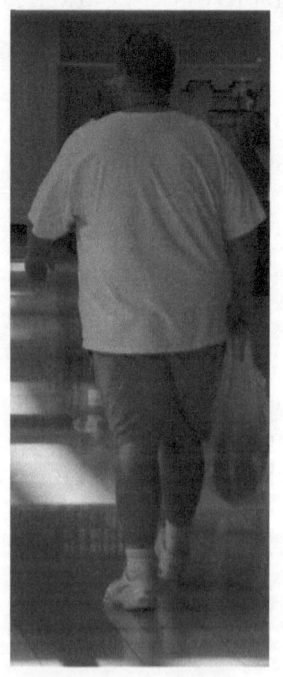
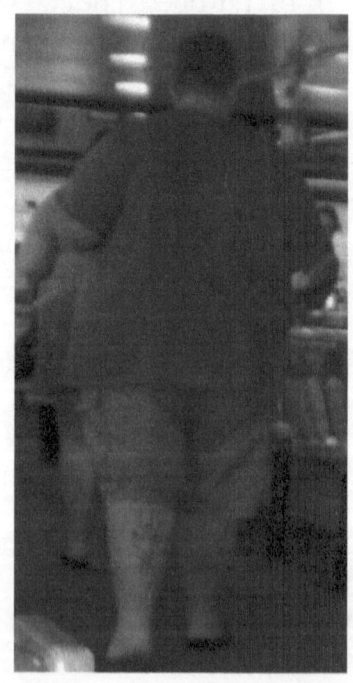

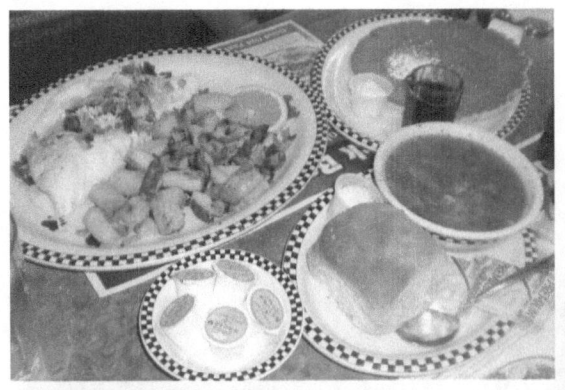

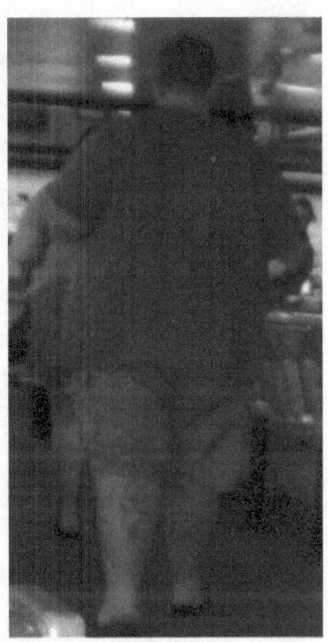

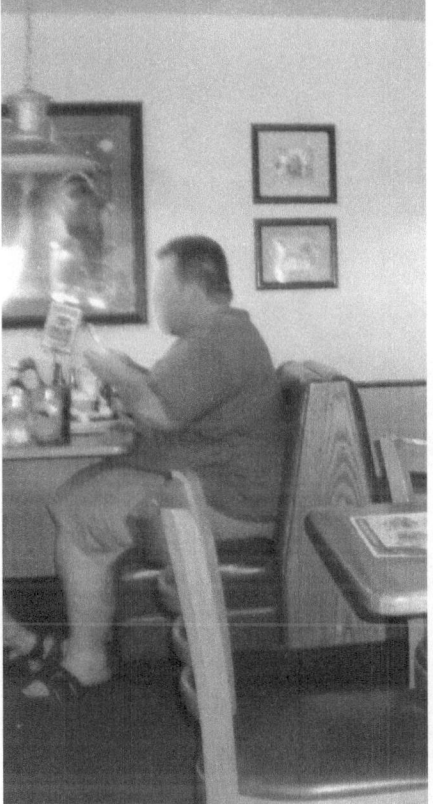

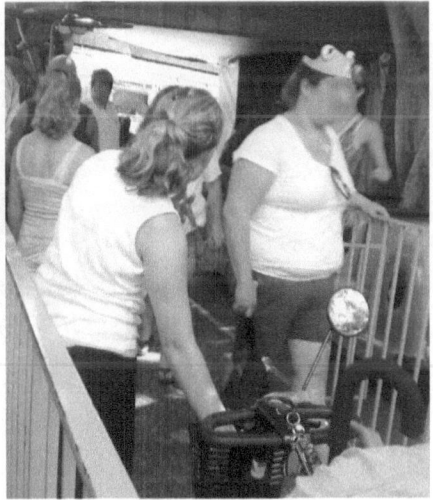

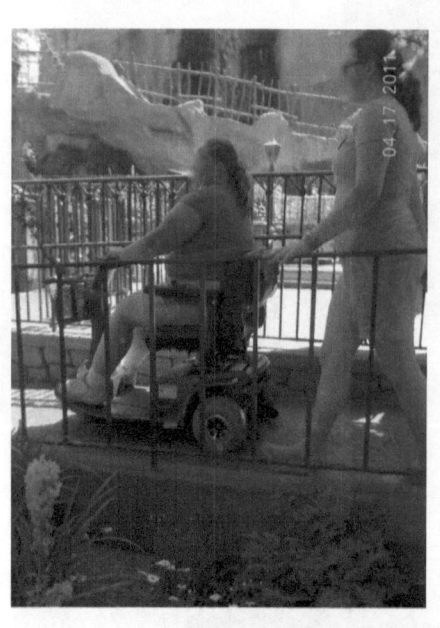

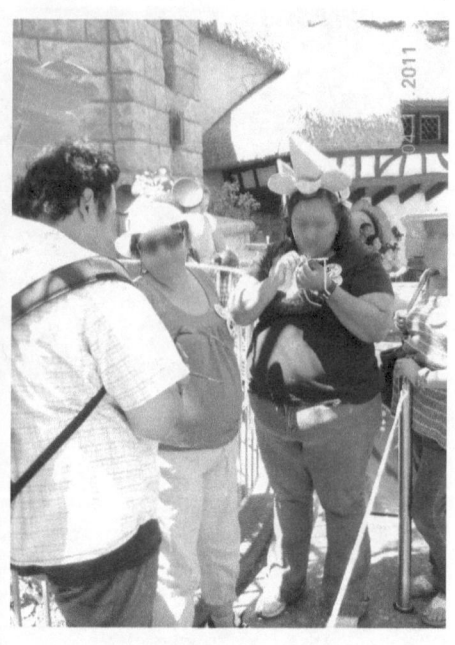

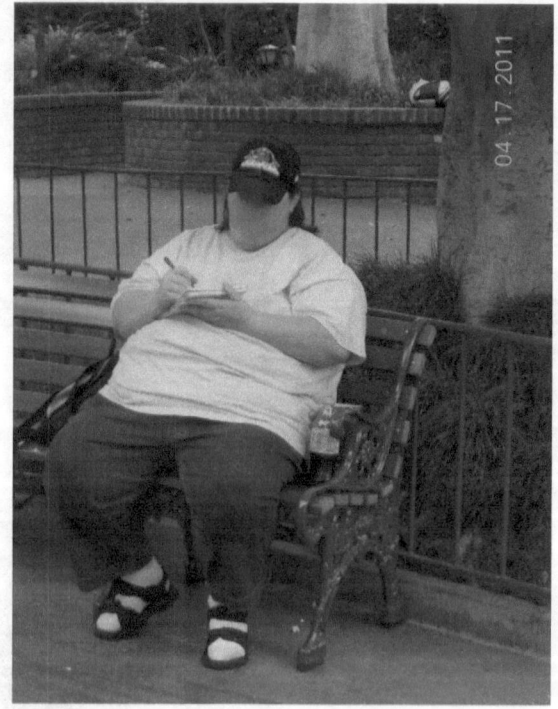

CHAPTER 3

Diseases and Medical Conditions Related to Obesity

31) A person with a normal weight is considered to carry 25 to 35 billion fat cells, but when the person is considered obese, the number of fat cells in the body is between 100 and 150 billion.

32) Researchers have proven that been obese is causative of developing diseases like a person with a normal weight is considered to carry 25 to 35 billion fat cells but hypertension, type 2 diabetes, cancer, stroke, and many others including gallstones.

33) Sexual abuse history is considered a risk to develop obesity later in life because of depression and lack of self-esteem.

34) Obese men have a risk of 25 to 30 percent of developing impotence and erectile dysfunction.

35) Obese women using oral contraceptives are more prone to get pregnant while taking the pill than women within their normal weight.

36) Seventy percent of heart disease in the United States is related directly to obesity. It is the number 1 cause of deaths in the world.

37) Obese people have more than a 40 percent chance to develop colon cancer than normal-weight people.

38) In the world actually there are one billion overweight people, and out of that billion, 300 million are clinically obese.

39)   Morbid obese is considered a person with a BMI of 40 or higher. Body mass index is the parameter used to measure obesity.

40)   Among other diseases, obese people are candidates to develop certain types of cancer, sleep apnea, high blood pressure, gallstones, and osteoarthritis. This means death and lack of quality of life.

41)   Metabolic syndrome is a condition that includes diabetes, obesity, high blood pressure, high triglycerides, and high blood cholesterol due to overweight.

42)   Severe obesity, meaning a BMI of >40, decreases life expectancy for ten years; less severe obesity (between 30 and 40) reduces life expectancy for an average of three years.

43)   An obese smoker has between four and five times more chances of early death; in the United States, 20 percent of obese adults are smokers.

44)   There is a link between vitamin D deficiency and obesity; the research shows that vitamin D lowers the concentration of hormone leptin.

45)   The hormone leptin is involved in the control or regulation of weight. Research shows that leptin sends a signal to the brain and lets it know when fat cells are satisfied.

46)   Let's be realistic: obesity is not only a cosmetic problem, it's an enormous hazard to our health. Obese and overweight people are twice as likely to develop high blood pressure and diabetes among other health problems.

47)   If the person has the extra weight concentrated around the waist, it is called "apple" shape, and they have more chances to develop health complications due to excess of weight than the people that have extra weight around the hips called "pear" shape.

Losing just 10 to 15 pounds will lower blood pressure and improve levels of cholesterol for an average of 10 percent.

48)   Of all the cases of type 2 diabetes, 80 percent of them are weight related. If you lose some weight and exercise more, you decrease your chances of developing type 2 diabetes.

49) Alcoholism is also related to obesity; some people just substitute one dependency for another. If there is history of alcoholism in the family, women are 50 percent more likely to develop obesity.

50) Eating in excess is an addiction, just like drugs or alcohol. Dr. William Philpot, MD, believes that food intake increases a substance called enkephalin, a narcotic produced by the body similar to opiates that are obtained externally.

51) People have a tendency to substitute food and use it as a drug, for example, wheat is the most substituted, and products that contain wheat like crackers, cakes, and cereals are the most used as drug of choice by the food addicts.

52) Hardening of arteries or atherosclerosis is ten times more prevalent in obese people than in people with a normal weight.

53) Sleep apnea is a condition that causes temporary stop of breathing while a person is sleeping. The fat around the neck of obese people put pressure on the air channel, making breathing more difficult. People with sleep apnea are sleepy during the day and may even have accidents because they fall to sleep anytime even when driving due to the lack of proper sleep. Just by losing 10 percent of your body weight, you decrease the chances of developing this condition.

54) Gallbladder is directly affected by obesity because it makes gallbladder to work harder to process fat. As many as 30 percent of gallbladder surgeries are due to obesity.

55) The excess of weight applies pressure to the inner part of the stomach which will send acid through the esophagus, and the person develops what is called gastroesophageal disease. If the person reduces weight, the pressure over the stomach is less, and the symptoms of reflux will improve.

56) People that are obese have greater chances to develop depression since obese people usually develop low self-esteem. By the same token, depressed people have greater chances of developing obesity due to lack of exercise and excessive eating as a result of their mental status.

57)   A person under stress has more chance to gain weight because he or she will eat more, faster, and inappropriate, so we can see that there is a tremendous link between stress and obesity, especially in the United States where people live under conditions more stressful than other countries.

58)   If we are under stress, the release of the hormone cortisol is higher. Cortisol is well-known to increase appetite and make people more anxious for sugary and fatty foods.

59)   Many people eat in excess food rich in fat and sugar because without being aware of it, they are trying to increase levels of serotonin in their body. Serotonin is a chemical known for making us feel good. This happens usually under stressful situations.

60)   Research shows that pregnant women that consumed a lot of excitotoxin-containing foods are at higher risk of having diabetic children than mothers that do not consume this type of foods.

61)   Studies show that obese pregnant women have higher risk of spontaneous loss.
        Couples that are obese (both) have to wait longer before conceiving a child, more or less three times longer than normal couples, and men that are obese have a higher chance of being infertile than men with a normal body weight.

62)   Obese mothers have a higher chance of giving birth to premature and smaller babies than women with normal weight.

63)   Some studies indicate that obese women have hormone imbalances that may result in decreasing the chances of fertilization and normal implantation of the baby.

64)   In just three years it will be possible to have a new drug for obese people called liraglutide that besides helping lose weight will lower bad cholesterol and raise good cholesterol, and the scientists in charge of the project affirm that it can even cure diabetes.

65)   If a person uses a lot of laxatives to try to lose weight, the digestion and absorption of food would be seriously affected, and the person may become anemic.

66) "Lack of the hormone thyroxin, from the thyroid gland in the neck, leads to a condition called cretinism in childhood or myxoedema in adult life, in which there is a general slowing of all processes in the organism. This condition leads to gain of weight."

67) Medical procedures like liposuction among teenagers have increased three times to five thousand per year.

68) If a woman substitutes a healthy serving of protein daily, she decreases her chances of getting coronary heart disease; for example, if instead of the red meat she eats a portion of nuts every day, her risk of developing coronary heart disease will be 30 percent lower.

69) If a woman is obese when she gets pregnant, the chances of having a baby with heart defects increase between 10 and 11 percent more than mothers with a normal weight.

70) Some researches link obesity to serious complications from the swine flu, including death. "We are surprised by the frequency of obesity among the severe cases that we have been tracking," said one of the CDC experts managing the outbreak of swine flu.

71) People who drink diet drinks and sodas don't lose weight, different studies show. In fact, the tendency is to slowly gain weight.

72) Drinking more than one soda daily (regular or diet) is linked to an increase in factors of risk for heart and coronary disease. Individuals drinking one or more sodas daily have a 49 percent higher risk of developing metabolic syndrome. This includes increase in waist circumference, high blood sugar and high cholesterol, high BMI, high triglycerides, and high blood pressure.

73) Twenty-nine percent of the obese people in the United States are so heavy and immobile that even committing suicide is not a viable option, since they are "physically unable to end their own fat lives."

74) Both obesity and drug addiction have been linked to a dysfunction in the brain reward system. In both cases,

overconsumption can trigger a gradual increase in the reward threshold, requiring more and more palatable high-fat food or reinforcing drug to satisfy the craving over time.

75)   Overeating is a disease of addiction, exactly like alcohol or drugs. The addiction to food is progressive, affecting the health and quality of life of the individuals addicted.

76)   The rates of obesity among children have tripled over the last thirty years.

Among married couples, the possibility of husband or wife becoming obese if the spouse becomes obese is 37 percent higher than couples with normal weights.

Among pairs of sisters and brothers, if one becomes obese, one will increase the chance of the other becoming obese by 41 percent.

77)   Obesity increases the chances of a person developing osteoarthritis because the joints' cartilages are under the pressure of the excess weight.

78)   Babies born to obese mothers have greater risk of developing asthma than babies born to normal-weight mothers.

79)   Based in recent studies, men that are obese one year before prostatic cancer is diagnosed are 2.5 times more likely than men with normal weight to die of prostatic cancer. The relationship between genitourinary cancer and obesity is more than impressive.

80)   Obesity also affects sexuality. In a study of 1,000 obese men, 50 percent of them had a decreased sexual desire, 42 percent felt they had difficulties performing sexually, and 41 percent just avoided any type of sexual contact.

81)   In a review of more than a one hundred research studies, scientists found that overweight and obese girls reach puberty earlier than girls with a normal weight.

82)   Bisphenol A (BPA) is a substance found in thermal paper. A recent study relates bisphenol A to obesity. We find BPA also in money in form of bills and receipts from cash registers.

83)   A recent study showed that women and men with a history of family alcoholism are 49 percent more likely to become

obese than members of families where alcoholism is not prevalent. Ironically, people with alcoholism problems seem to keep a normal weight.

84) Newborns that are breast-fed are less likely to become obese as they grow older than babies that are not breast-fed as they get older, and mothers who breast-feed return to prepregnancy weight easier than mothers who don't breast-feed.

85) Being fat, overweight or obese, increases the chances of developing restless leg syndrome (RLS), a disorder that causes people to feel the need to keep moving their legs, especially when they are lying down. Restless leg syndrome has an impact on sleep and quality of life.

86) A study in Israel found that obese children are more prone to develop attention-deficit/hyperactivity disorder. It may be that excessive eating is a psychological response to the stress of being ADHD.

87) Hypertension, until recently virtually unseen in young people, now strikes an estimated 4.5 percent of obese school-age children.

88) A team of researchers evaluated the relationship between depression and obesity over time and found out that there is a bidirectional relationship because an obese person has a 55 percent increased chance of developing depression, and depressed persons have a 58 percent increased risk of becoming obese.

89) Researchers from St. Louis University in Missouri found that children who get their *tonsils* removed gain more weight after the operation than children who don't have the operation. Increase in weight could be seen up to seven years after the procedure.

90) Ghrelin has been identified as the first circulating hunger hormone. Ghrelin levels get higher before meals and get lower after meals.

91) Resveratrol is a compound present in grapes and red wine. This substance reduces the amount of fat cells and is used to prevent and treat obesity. This finding is consistent with

the hypothesis that resveratrol in wine explains the French paradox, the fact that French people eat a diet rich in fats but have a low incidence of heart disease.

92) A team of American researchers at Texas A and M University found out that the amino acid arginine helps fight obesity in humans. The foods that contain arginine are seafoods, watermelon, nuts, seeds, meats, rice, and soy.

93) Polycystic ovary syndrome is a condition that affects 10 percent of women eighteen to forty years old. This condition is a common cause of infertility. Recent studies have shown that polycystic ovary syndrome and obesity are related, the more obese the more likely the women are to develop this syndrome and to have fertility problems.

94) Obstructive sleep apnea is a syndrome that results in excessive daytime sleepiness. It increases the chances of motor vehicle accidents and is very common among truck drivers. Approximately 4 million commercial drivers in the United States are expected to have this condition. The leading fact for apnea is obesity, and truck drivers with sleep apnea have up to seven times more chances of being involved in a vehicle crash than drivers with a normal weight.

95) A 10-kilogram weight loss can produce a 15-percent decrease in the LDL (bad cholesterol) and an increase of 8 percent in HDL (good cholesterol).

A child that is overweight or obese is at 75 percent risk of becoming overweight or obese as an adult, which among other conditions can increase the risk of cancer, diabetes, and heart disease.

96) Children that are obese have an increased risk of loosening of teeth (periodontoclasia) because the heavier or more obese the child is, the higher the incidence of caries on his/her teeth.

97) Sleep apnea is a type of sleep disorder that is directly related to obesity because the fat tissue around the neck obstructs the airway pass and causes pauses during the sleep. The fatter you are, the higher the chances of developing apnea. Studies demonstrate also a relationship between apnea and heart disease.

98)   Cortisol is a hormone involved in the body's response to stress. When the stress goes up, the levels of cortisol go up. Research demonstrates that obese people have higher levels of cortisol in blood than normal-weight people. If you are under stress often, your chances of getting obese are higher than people that are not under stress.

99)   Obese people that underwent bariatric surgery and lost significant weight reduced their risk of dying by nearly 50 percent. Morbid obese people carry a double chance of risk of dying as a result to complications related to their weight including heart disease, diabetes, high blood pressure, etc.

100)   A big waist nearly doubles the risk of a person's early death from causes like cancer, heart disease, diabetes, and respiratory illness, and a big waist also increases the risk of death even in people that are not overweight.

101)   According to new estimates, every year 124,000 new cancers in Europe are caused by overweight and obesity. The highest number was found in women living in Central Europe such as Bulgaria, Slovenia, and Latvia.

102)   Obese men should lose weight if they want to have children because obesity is linked to a lower volume of semen and a higher percent of abnormal sperm.

103)   In a couple, if both partners are obese or overweight, they are more likely to wait longer before conceiving a child. If both partners are obese, the wait before conceiving a child is three times higher than in couples with normal weights.

104)   New research from the Baylor College of Medicine in Houston, Texas, suggests that women who are overweight or obese before and during their pregnancy will pass on their obesity to their unborn child.

105)   The World Health Organization forecasts that by the year 2015, which is only four years away, the number of clinically obese people in the world will reach 700 million people.

106)   A study from Boston University concludes that obese people find it harder to fight infections due to a weakened immune system.

107)   Researchers from the FDA (Food and Drug Administration) has given approval for a trial involving injection lypolosis which has become commonly known as fat dissolving. Basically, various compounds are injected into the subcutaneous fat in certain parts of the body where there is an unwanted local accumulation of fat. The fat is broken down and excreted by the body.

108)   A report from the European Union's statistical office concludes that 23 percent of the British women are clinically obese. According to medical sources, being obese can take around nine years off your life and can lead to a host of health complications such as diabetes, heart disease, stroke, infertility, and depression among others.

109)   A stomach pacemaker is a device that consists of a stimulator and a sensor surgically implanted onto the stomach. The stimulator sends out electrical pulses meant to trick the stomach and brain into thinking that the body is full. The stomach pacemaker is available for sale in Europe and is one the last developments to fight obesity.

110)   A study of the two most popular weight-loss surgeries found obese diabetics who had gastric bypass surgery lost 64 percent of their excess weight after a year compared with 37 percent in those treated with the Lap-Band device.

111)   A leading health expert has come out publicly and said that he thinks teenagers and perhaps even children should be fitted with gastric bands. Professor Nick Finer of University College Hospital is an expert in obesity and earlier in the year told the Royal Society of Medicine that severely obese children should be permitted to undergo bariatric surgery, such as gastric banding. He says that the excess of fat can affect the blood vessels in children as young as six years old.

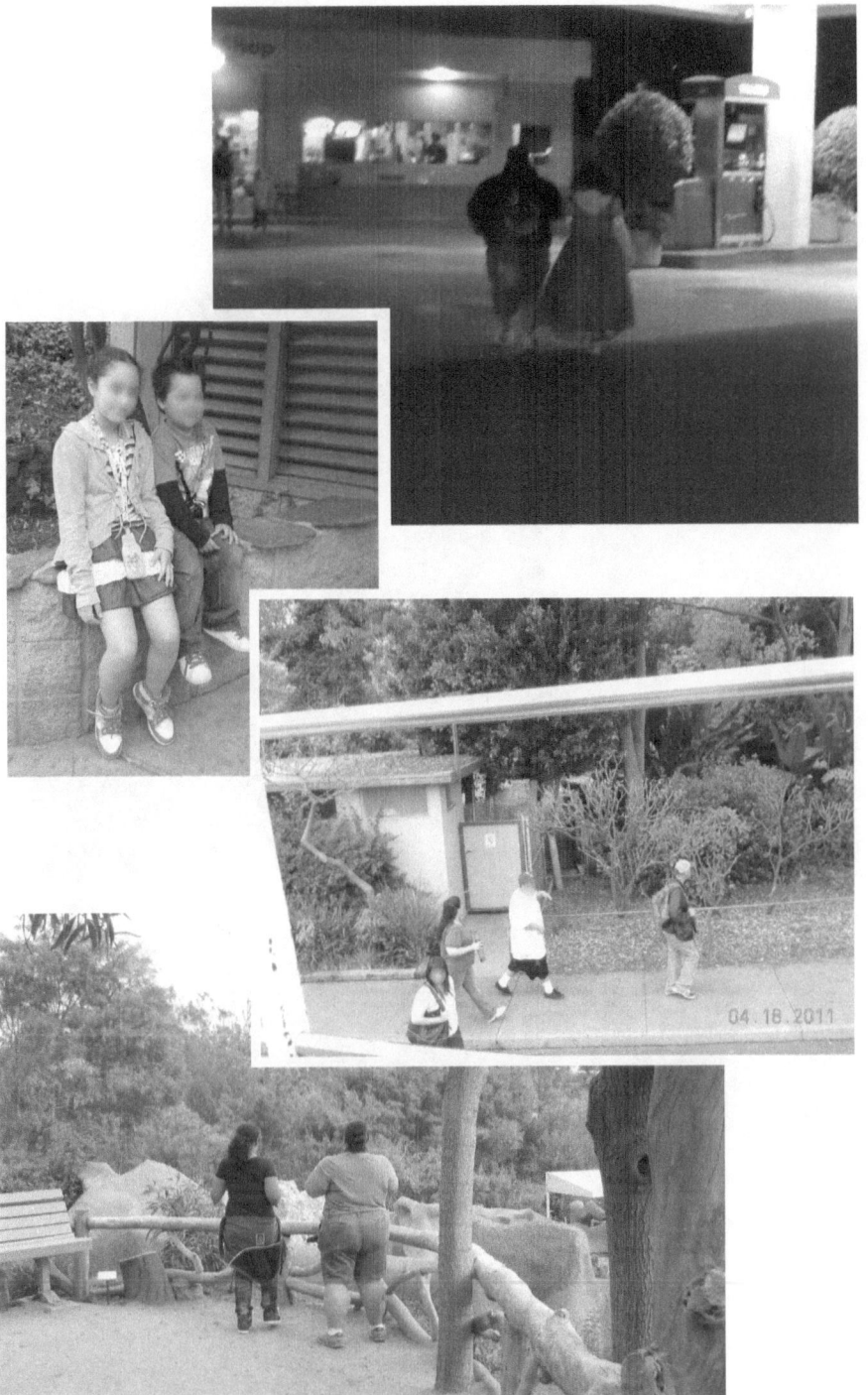

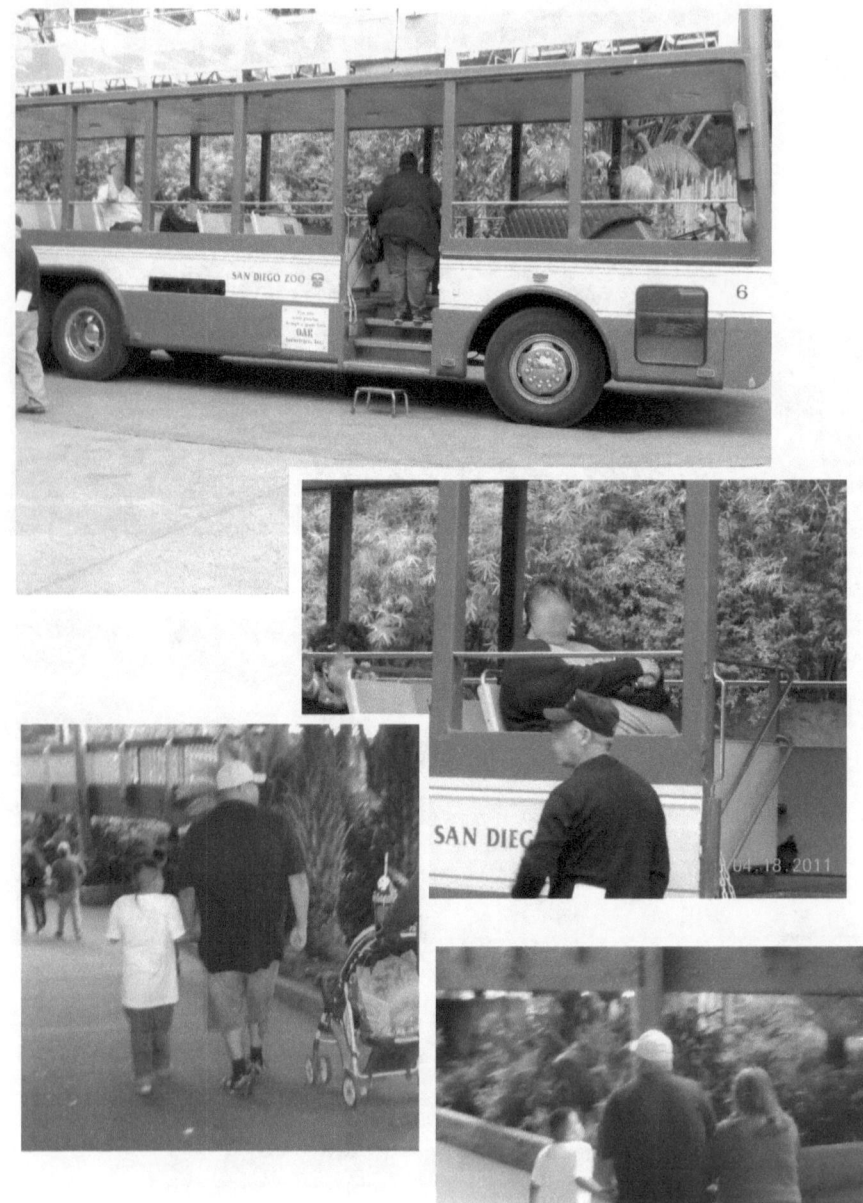

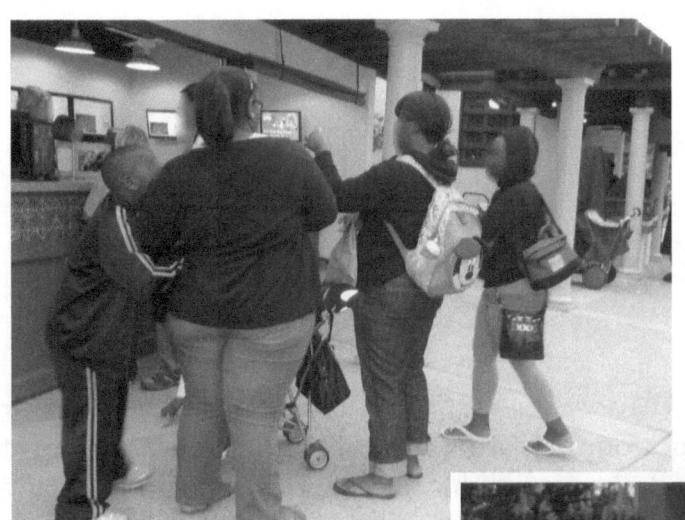

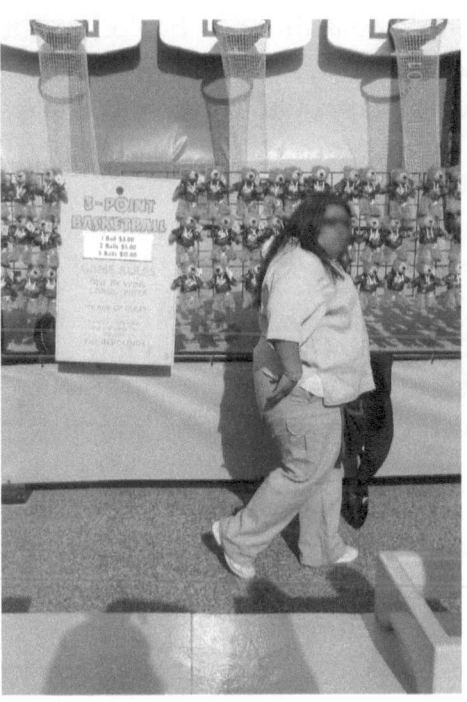

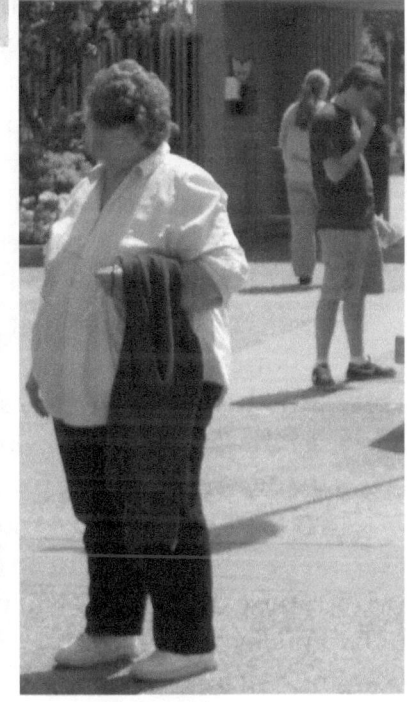

CHAPTER 4

Curiosities and Facts

112) Santa Claus was a fat, drunken, reckless menace to society. A team from Monash University in Melbourne has written in the *British Journal* that Santa Claus should be rebranded for a more health-conscious age. They believe images of him in advertising should be regulated because of the potentially harmful messages he conveys.

113) A recent study by Harvard researchers in which they added a 35 percent tax to sugary sodas sold in a cafeteria found that sales of sugar-sweetened sodas dropped by 26 percent and that people tended to replace those drinks with soda or coffee. This means that a food tax could trim some people's calorie intake.

114) Run by the United States Department of Agriculture, the *Apps for Healthy Kids* competition challenges software developers to develop engaging tools and games that help kids and their parents to eat better and be more physically active.

115) The latest in weight loss treatment for the morbidly obese comes in the form of a new device called the Ability System, an electronic implant which is inserted into the body below the ribs and controls eating behavior.

116) Researchers at Oxford University have found a relationship between fat mass, excess weight, and a gene that is associated directly with obesity—the FTO gene. The gene appears to be responsible for obesity and overeating.

117) Major Bloomberg of New York City is asking permission to ban the purchasing of soda and sugary drinks using food

stamps. The value of the food stamps would remain the same meaning that there would be more money spent on nutritious food in New York City.

118) Some vegetables contain fermentable carbohydrates that activate hormones in the gut which suppress appetite, for example, asparagus, artichokes, garlic, and chicory.

119) Researchers from University College of London believe that banning junk food ads could cut rates of childhood obesity by as much as 14 percent. The report concluded that food advertising had an unhealthy impact of how children aged between six and eleven eat.

120) A new test scheme in England called Weight Wins has shown that dieters who are paid to lose weight are far more likely to succeed than those who are not. Dieters sign for a pound-for-pound scheme where they get paid for every pound they lose and then are given a cash bonus after a certain number of months in the program if they manage to keep the weight off.

121) According to Pennsylvania State University researchers, adding pureed vegetable to entrees reduces the number of calories the meals contain without sacrificing taste and adding fiber and vitamins to the diet.

122) By cutting back 360 calories each day, a person could lose one pound of body fat in about ten days.

123) Some chemically enhanced caramel food coloring used in widely consumed cola drinks could cause cancer and should be banned; a U.S. consumer advocacy group urged the Food and Drug Administration. Pure caramel is made from melted sugar, but two other versions approved to color food products include the chemical ammonia which produces cancer in humans.

124) The Agriculture Department in the United States has approved three more genetically engineered crops in 2011, and the Food and Drug Administration could approve fast-growing genetically modified fish (salmon) for human consumption in the next two or three months.

125)   Rhythm Pharmaceuticals, a startup company in Boston, tested its experimental diet drug on some of the Oregon research monkeys. After eight weeks, the animals reduced 40 percent of their food intake and lost 13 percent of their weight without apparent heart problems. The monkeys serve as useful models because they resemble humans more than laboratory rats do, not only physiologically but in some of their feeding habits.

126)   Airlines are spending $275 million buying 350 million gallons of additional fuel to compensate for the passengers' extra weight that are all obese.

127)   Males and females that lost 10 percent of their weight had an increase in the quality of their sexual life.

128)   Researchers found out that 35 percent of our caloric intake every day comes from foods bought in restaurants (incredible).

129)   The biggest epidemic in children in this century is obesity, and in almost all the world, the obesity rate among children is getting higher and in history the worst epidemic of all.

130)   Studies show that people are willing to give up a year of their life instead of being obese; other people are willing to become blind or lose a limb (leg or arm) due to lack of self-esteem and depression.

131)   In the United States, the obesity rate is now twice than in 1980. At that time, there were 150 million, and now the number is 300 million.

132)   When you use a credit card to pay at the restaurant, you are prone to overspend and order more food than when you use cash to pay for it.

133)   A person is considered obese when his/her body mass index is 30 or greater.
        The direct cost of obesity in the United States is $147 billion.
        Only 2 percent of the children in the Unites States eat healthy by the FDA (Food and Drug Administration) standards.

134)   The average child in this country spends an average of four hours daily in front of the television.

135) It is estimated that by the age of five, a child is exposed to twenty thousand food commercials.

136) The average cost for bariatric surgery is $30,000 for a child and $38,000 for an adult. If you invest $35,000 (at 5 percent interest), after forty years, you will have more than $3 million in your account.

137) Obese people that drive spend about $40 more for gasoline per year.
For an obese person, life insurance is $110 more expensive than for a thin person.

138) To lose 1 pound of weight, a person needs to burn 3,500 calories, that is about 5 hours on the treadmill at a speed of 7 miles per hour.

139) For an obese person, the costs of medical insurance are more or less $1,000 more expensive than for a person that is not overweight.

140) Many companies in the United States do not build plants in the states with high prevalence of obese people, in part due to the high cost in health insurance and loss of work due to diseases related to obesity.

141) Mississippi is the number 1 state in obesity in the United States, and Colorado is the state with less number of overweight and obese people.

142) Employers have three main reasons to not hire an obese person: costs of health insurance, limitations to perform physical activities, and the image of the business. (Being obese means death!)

143) Prospective obese employees are seen as less active workers by employers, so it is harder to get a job.

144) For an obese person, it is extremely difficult to get a promotion at work; and they are placed mainly in positions where they don't have close contact with the customer, for example, obese people are good candidates to work in a call center because of the personal appreciation common to an obese person.

145) Some airlines have weight restrictions for flight attendants but not for pilots because pilots hardly have any contact with passengers even if they are obese.

If we consider the data of the obesity in the United States, we find that it is twice than in 1970.

146)   The tangible cost in health and work-related expenses for an obese woman is $4,800 more per year than a woman with a normal weight.

Paying with credit cards at restaurants increases the amount of food that is ordered, and people have the tendency to overeat if they are paying with plastic instead of cash. Even credit cards have an impact on obesity.

147)   If the actual trend in obesity continues, this will be the first generation with a reduced life expectancy in history of humanity. (We are killing each other and our kids and even our pets, not through terrorism, but through eating.)

148)   Due to the number of overweight and obese babies, the makers of car seats for infants are increasing the size of such seats to accommodate bigger babies. Can you believe that?

149)   Japan is the country in the world with less obese people, and Samoa is the country with the higher rate of overweight and obese citizens.

150)   The federal government has valued life of a human being through three different agencies:

EPA (Environmental Protection Agency): $9.1 million
FDA (Food and Drug Administration): $7.9 million
DT (Department of Transportation): $6 million

151)   In 2010 the cost of obesity-related deaths is extremely high by any of the three standards if we consider the number of the United States citizens that are obese. This is the worst epidemic known to humankind—not the plague, not terrorism, not drugs, not war, but eating in excess.

152)   Some societies of the Pacific practice fattening routines to make women more attractive and men stronger. This is the case in places like Tahiti and Nauru.

If you tried to control your eating and you are unable to or if you eat when you are under stress or strong emotions or if you induce vomiting after overeating, most probably you are a food addict.

153) The body mass index (BMI) is just a mathematical formula that divides your body weight in kilograms by your height in meters (squared).

154) A good nutrition early on life is very important in the development of parts of the brain that regulate weight.

155) The price of fruits and vegetables increased 50 percent between 1982 and 2008 (real cost). On the other hand, fast food got cheaper and more readily available.

156) In 2008 during the recession crisis, the fast-food chains outperformed the standard and poor index because people were consuming less expensive food regardless of the quality.

157) During economic stress situations, the obesity rate has a tendency to increase due to the fact that it leaves almost no time for outdoor activities, homemade meals, and attendance to gyms and spas will most likely decline.

158) Experts estimate that more than 50 percent of dogs in the United States are overweight or obese, that means more or less 40 million dogs are obese or overweight in this country.

159) The problem of obesity is reaching our pets to the point that last year two drugs were approved for use in canine obesity.

160) Stevia is a species of herb that is three hundred times sweeter than sugar. In Japan, it is used since sixty years ago. It is completely natural, and so far, no side effects were found due to the use of stevia as a sweetener. In the United States, the use of stevia was approved in 2008, but there is still a long way to go to compete with the conventional sweeteners (nonnatural). Japan is the country with the lowest obesity rate in the world.

161) You should not allow yourself to become extremely hungry because it is harder to make rational decisions about what to eat, and because if you skip meals, your glucose level in blood will be low, and you will become more anxious about eating. Experts recommend never skip meals.

162) Size of portions are very important, and if you are under stress, you have the tendency to eat larger portions.

163) Always try to engage in activities that decrease stress like walking, biking, swimming, any type of exercise, or meditation. Try to spend time with friends, and if necessary, look for a specialist to get help managing your stress levels.

164) Children that are obese or overweight have more difficulty playing sports and taking part in school activities, and they are very prone to depression.

165) Some experts believe that the main reason for the enormous increase in obesity is the sedentary way of life adopted by this generation. According to Centers for Disease Control and Prevention, "between 1970 and 2000 the average American man increased his caloric intake by 168 calories a day (17 pounds a year) while the average woman added 335 calories a day."

166) Media also plays an important role in the development of this pandemic of obesity, for example, actors, sports stars, even politicians endorse junk foods like French fries. We need to understand that children take these celebrities as role models!

167) Computer games, television shows, and most of the electronic gadgets are used by children who are spending more time inside the house eating and not spending that excess caloric intake.

168) On top of the Internet, cell phones, etc., our children also face academic duties like homework, tests, grades, making it more difficult for them to find the time to exercise.

169) Some people overeat because they firmly believe that it is immoral to throw away food. Others with inferiority complexes just eat and eat to develop a feeling of security.

170) If we examine the historic background of the United States, we find since the colonies an obsession with food, we got to the point of industrial revolution. We had the machinery and tools to make food more abundant and less expensive, and we had excess crops that provided farmers with extra

money. With that extra money, eating out began to be more and more common and obesity more and more rampant.

171) Overweight people and obese people have less chance to get accepted by prestigious colleges and universities. That is another limitation in the life of an obese person.

172) Some parents, especially minorities, have the tendency to make children eat even when they are not hungry. This promotes an excessive intake of calories and the possible development of obesity at an early age, plus making a child to finish up all the food on his/her plate is another factor that contributes to obesity.

173) Research tells us that food is a substitute for love: ice cream, candies, even chocolate are usually presents for the ones we love as a signal of love.

174) Different studies prove that there is a direct relationship between obesity and the frequency of hospitalizations. The length of hospitalization is in an average thirty-six hours longer in an obese person than in a person that is thin.

175) In England, five thousand nurses are undergoing back pain treatment due to patients' obesity and the effort needed to move them.

176) Morbid obese people pay as much as twice in medical care than people considered in a normal weight.

177) The indirect costs of obesity, like employee absenteeism or showing to work ill or performing less than the normal, is more than $73 billion. This added to the direct costs which gives us more than $300 billion per year.

178) Obese people lose an average of six days of work every year due to conditions related to the excess of weight more than people with a normal weight.

179) In a study covered by natural news, researchers found that obesity-related expenses cost more than $344 billion a year. When combined with current productivity loss figures, total obesity-related cost approached nearly half trillion dollars a year.

180) In 2006, the costs related to obesity made up for 9 percent of all the medical expenses in this country.

181)   One billion dollars in 100 bills is the equivalent of the height of half of the Empire State Building, so to keep $300 billion in $100 bills, we will need 150 buildings like the Empire State Building! That is a lot of space!

182)   Excitotoxins are substances that overstimulate neurons, getting them to the point of cell death. Many chemicals like aspartame and monosodium glutamate are used routinely in fried foods and snacks. Some studies done in animals prove that monosodium glutamate is linked to lesions in the hypothalamus that causes many health problems including overweight, short stature, and fertility problems. In most of the chips and other fried foods, monosodium glutamate is used.

183)   When obesity is caused from exposure to exitotoxins, the task of losing weight is especially difficult because it does not appear to be related to the food intake. This may be a reason why some people find especially difficult to diet successfully.
        Since humans lack a barrier in the hypothalamus, the exposure to excitotoxins is much more dangerous than animals.

184)   In developed countries, because of different reasons, women have the tendency to have babies later in life (older than thirty-five). If a woman is obese and above thirty years old, the chances of getting pregnant are reduced.

185)   Obesity is a condition that includes excess of adipose tissue volume. People can develop obesity without necessarily being overweight, and some overweight people, especially weight lifters, can be overweight and not obese.

186)   To measure the body fatness, the most accurate method is called dual-energy x-ray absorptiometry (dexa). It uses two x-ray beams with different intensities as both move through an individual body.

187)   Obesity is becoming such a problem in the United States that police officers are failing their physicals. Police officers and firefighters are seen by children as an example. If they see obese officers, the tendency to accept that condition is

higher, making it more difficult to control the epidemic of obesity.

188) The owners of theaters are replacing the seats to fit the big rear ends of obese people. Seats used to be 17 to 20 inches in wide. The new seats start at 19 inches! On top theater environment makes people overeat, especially foods high in fats and low in nutritional value, for example, popcorn can get up to 1,200 calories per serving.

189) The famous actor Marlon Brando suffered from obesity to the point that during the making of One-Eyed Jacks, his clothing had to be made of plastic elastic material. The weight was so high that even with the elastic clothing he did split eighteen pairs of pants!

190) The actress Kristie Allen used to drink fourteen sodas daily, and she was depressed all the time; finally, she was able to lose weight and partially recovered her shape.

191) Carol Yeager got to weigh 1,200 pounds because of her obesity. She required between 17 and 20 firefighters to carry and help her to go to the hospital. She died at thirty-four.

192) Some morbid obese people lack at least a set of genes, at least 7 percent of morbid obese people are born without 30 genes of the estimated 30,000 genes in human genetic structure.

193) The Last Supper of da Vinci is very famous because it presents an image of Christ and his twelve apostles, eating their last dinner together. Experts in computer analysis have proven after analyzing more than fifty paintings that the main meals, plates, bread sizes have keep growing through the time; so the size of portions for the Last Supper in 2011 would be 68 percent bigger, demonstrating that the size of portions also is a big problem that leads to obesity.

194) Fear of not getting enough food leads some people, who have once been hungry, to overeat whenever there is a chance, and people that have gone hungry during childhood never quite lose the fear of hunger and may tend to overeat when they have become rich. This accounts for the traditional, portly figure of the self-made man.

195)   Since obesity may be triggered by emotional facts, hypnosis is used with some success in some obesity cases.

196)   Our body cannot make some proteins, they need to be in our food. Vitamin C also is not produced by the body but provided by our diet.

197)   Long time ago in Australia, the missionaries were having a lot of troubles trying to stop cannibalism among aborigines, especially when the deceased was fat. When a thin man died, it was easy to stop cannibalism; but when a fat person died, missionaries had to guard the cadaver because sometimes the aborigines ate the body days or weeks after death. (This is to show the attraction that people have for fatty foods.)

198)   Exercise increases calorie expenditure and also makes the organism to use the stored fat, so let's exercise!

199)   Every month, 9 of 10 American children visit fast-food restaurants, making easier the development of obesity.

200)   The first printed reference to hamburgers was published by *Los Angeles Times* in 1894.

201)   Youngsters consume approximately 66 gallons of soda per year, every soda has a high content of sugar, and drinking so many of the soft drinks is a big factor in this obesity pandemic.

202)   In the year 2004, Americans ate more than 7 billion pounds of potatoes, mainly fried.

203)   In the United States, there are more than 325,000 fast-food restaurants.

204)   Recently in Ontario, Canada, a judge took away a child from her obese mother because he firmly believed that an obese mother was causing an overweight problem for the child, and the judge was very concerned about the girl's medical problems.

205)   At the end of his life, the great Elvis Presley was consuming daily more or less 85,000 calories. His favorite food was a sandwich with a pound of bacon, a jar of peanut butter, and a pint of grape jelly. A sandwich like that was enough to feed eight people. Elvis kept a chef 24/7 to cook anything

he wanted besides the sandwiches, including French fries, cookies, pies, etc.

206) In Mexico, there is a morbid obese man that got to weigh 1,200 pounds. Newborn elephants weight between 165 and 255 pounds, so this man weighed the equivalent to five or six baby elephants. After doing a diet, he lost 400 pounds but still is unable to walk and spends his days in a specially designed industrial-sized bed. Interesting enough, this man does not have diabetes, heart disease, or high triglycerides! There is no explanation for this.

207) Twenty years ago in New York, Michael Hebranko hold the title of the heaviest man in the world at 1,100 pounds. He could eat 24 eggs or 3 dozen pork chops or 24 bagels at one time with two pounds of cream cheese. He lost 900 pounds in less than two years, and he became successful in his dieting; but his 200 pounds only lasted seven years, and Hebranko was up to 1,000 pounds.

208) In 2006, a group of researchers followed 2,000 low-income children in twenty-six cities, and their findings were that 33.3 percent were obese before the age of four years. Hispanics were the most affected ethnic group.

209) The consumption of sodas has increased 300 percent in the last two decades; that increase is one of the reasons for the obesity pandemic in 2010.
Twenty-five percent of all the vegetables consumed in the United States are French fries or chips.

210) Our generation ingests 20 percent more calories than the previous generation; those calories come mainly from fats (63 percent), sugar, and grains.
Twenty-five percent of teenagers drink an average of four soft drinks daily that is the equivalent of an extra meal.

211) Nine out of ten food commercials during Saturday morning's television programming are for foods of poor nutrition, according to a study by the University of Minnesota.

212) The average weight for U.S. citizens increased 9 pounds between the year 1991 and 2000.

213)   Virgin Atlantic paid Barbara Hewson from Wales the equivalent of $24,100 in 2002 as compensation after she was squashed by an obese person sitting next to her on a transatlantic flight. Barbara suffered a blood clot in her chest, torn leg muscles, and acute sciatica and was bedridden for a month.

214)   Active transportation, transit systems are linked to less obesity rates, and countries like the United States that lack mass transit infrastructure are linked to higher overweight and obesity rates.

215)   Sixty percent of the pets in the United States are overweight or obese. The average dog owner spends between $250 and $300 a year on dog food. The cat owners spend a little less, $190 to $200 per year.

216)   Pet obesity can be expensive. Only in 2009, there were more than $17 million in claims to insurance companies to treat problems directly linked to pets' obesity.

217)   In Brazil, a country known by the "Girl of Ipanema," obesity is causing a lot of problems to the point that 25 percent of hospital beds are taken by people suffering weight-linked problems such as back surgeries, infarcts, replacement of hip or shoulders. If this obesity trend continues, in a few years we will have the "Fat Girl of Ipanema."

218)   For regular soda drinkers, the chance of becoming obese or overweight increases 48 percent if they drink more than two 12-ounce can of soda daily. For diet soda drinkers, the chance of getting obese or overweight was 58 percent for more than 2 cans daily.

219)   Some insurance industry analysts in the United States want to charge obese people with higher premiums; this can be seen by the people affected as a discriminatory practice. Other analysts suggest a federal tax credit for people that keep a normal weight.

220)   Obesity and overweight are linked to low levels of physical activity and low self-esteem; both factors can trigger depression.

221) There is a link between education and obesity, for example, women that hold a college degree are less likely to become obese than women that are less educated. Twenty-four percent of women with a four-year college degree are overweight or obese; this is lower than the 45 percent of women with high school education only.

200) Thirty-five million dogs and fifty-four million cats are estimated overweight or obese in the United States.

222) Surgeon General Richard Carmona says that obesity is a greater threat for the United States than terrorism.

223) Mike Huckabee, a Republican ex-Arkansas governor, wants to experiment with a system in which food stamps would be worth more if they were spent on healthy purchases like fruits and vegetables.

224) The top 5 countries with the higher rate of male obesity in the world are as follows: (1) Nauru, (2) Cook Islands, (3) Micronesia, (4) Tonga, and (5) the United States of America.

225) By 2018, in the United States, the expenses related directly to obesity are expected to account for more than 21 percent of the nation's health care spending.

226) Women are more likely to be obese than men in all groups of age.

The Framingham health study collected data from a group of 12,000 individuals, and the report documented, among other findings, the fact that if a person became obese, his or her friends had 57 percent higher chance of becoming obese also. If the friendship was a close one and considered mutual by both parties, that risk jumped to 171 percent!

227) In 2004, the Federal Aviation Administration increased its estimated weight of the average male in the United States from 170 to 184 pounds.

228) If the total of the morbid obese people of the U.S. lived in one state, it would be the state number 12 in population with more people than Virginia.

229)   The Pima Indians in Arizona developed high blood pressure, high blood sugar, and of course obesity after changing to the Western lifestyle.

230)   A study published in the *Archives of Pediatrics and Adolescent Medicine* found that three—to five-year-olds preferred *anything* wrapped in a McDonald's label to plain white paper.

231)   Only 20 percent of military aged Americans can join the military; the other 80 percent is just too fat to serve. Since 2005, the military rejected 48,000 recruits because of obesity, that figure is higher than all the troops fighting in Afghanistan.

232)   "A recent study by Wayne State University of 8,000 American infants revealed the following: 31.9 percent of 9 months old were obese or at risk of obesity; 34.3 percent of 2 years old were obese or at risk of becoming obese; 17 percent of the infants were obese at 9 months rising to 20 percent at two years; 44 percent of the infants that were obese at 9 months remained obese at 2 years. Hispanic and low-income children were at greater risk for weight status gain."

233)   "All indications are that this generation of children will grow into the fattest generation in the United States' history, and experts believe that next generation will be fatter and less fit than this generation."

234)   The number of states where adult obesity exceeds 30 percent doubled in the past year in the United States going from four to eight were Alabama, Kentucky, Oklahoma, Mississippi, West Virginia, Tennessee, Arkansas, and Louisiana.
        Adult obesity in Afro-Americans is 40 percent in 9 states, 35 percent in 34 states, and 30 percent in 43 states of the United States.

235)   Almost everybody remembers recent headlines about a forty-two-year-old woman in New Jersey who is trying to become the fattest woman on earth. While she only weighs 600 pounds, she is hoping to get to 1,000 pounds. People like this are called "gainers"—people that fantasize about becoming fat. There is a large sexual component to gainer culture with

many individuals being fat fetishists or adipophiles, meaning people that find fatness sexually attractive.

236) A large scale study at Case Western Reserve University (more than 68,000 women) found that those who sleep less than five hours a night gain more weight over time than those who sleep seven hours a night. Lack of enough sleep is another factor that increases the risks of becoming obese.

237) The lightest sleepers that only sleep from two to four hours per night are 68 percent more likely to become obese than people who sleep eight hours.

The painting of a morbid obese figure by Lucian Freud lying over a floral couch sold for $33.6 million, this is the highest price paid for an artwork by a living artist.

238) More than half of the United States' adults don't engage in regular exercise. Just 30 minutes of daily exercise can lower the risk of obesity and all the diseases linked to this condition.

239) Employers who are willing to promote health and prevention also get big rewards. For every dollar spent in programs to reduce obesity; they get an investment return of $1.50 to $3.50 in savings related to health care.

240) Four states and at least 15 local districts in the United States have passed legislation requiring fast-food restaurants to include calorie counts on menu, and the same measure has been introduced in 26 more states and in congress.

241) According to 2004 report by the Institute of Medicine Committee on Prevention of Obesity in Children and Youth, approximately 9 million American children over six years of age are considered obese, and many experts consider that the number is a lot higher.

242) *Girls on the Run*, a twelve-week program, aimed at third to fifth grade girls to combine training for a five-kilometer run with life skills development and lessons to enhance self-esteem, all of which can help reduce to prevent obesity. The program is active in more than 120 U.S. and Canada cities.

243) The giant food and beverage company, PepsiCo, has undertaken several initiatives to promote health and fitness including the *Smart Spot* program in which a symbol on a product's packaging identifies it as a healthy choice.

244) *America on the Move* is a program designed to encourage people of all ages to slowly make increases in walking and small decreases in intake of calories to prevent overweight and improve fitness. This program is designed to work at the local, state, and national levels.

245) In a study of two hundred neighborhoods, there were three times as many supermarkets in wealthy neighborhoods as in poor neighborhoods. This fact leaves fast-food places as the most convenient food option for many poor families. Obesity is linked directly to fast-food restaurants.

246) One of every four children does not participate in any free time physical activity, and 90 percent of elementary schools don't have daily exercise classes. Less than 25 percent of high school students in the United States take daily exercise classes.

247) There is a number of psychological effects that come with being overweight or obese. According to an American research, obese children consider their quality of life as being at the same level as those children suffering from cancer.

248) Obese people have problems finding clothing. Finding large sizes is very difficult, and if they find the right size, then most probably it will not be the latest style, and the price is going to be higher than regular size clothing.

249) Young people at the age of 6 are prejudiced against obesity and overweight. Children at the age of seven consider fat children as lazy, liars, ugly, or even stupid.

250) The pressure on young women to look like supermodels can result in weight problems because starving diet can have the opposite effect since after a period of dieting you will regain the weight after starting eating like before the diet.

251) The human cost of overweight and obesity in England is 18 million sick days a year, 30,000 deaths a year which result

in 10,000 lost years of working life—a life span which is shortened by approximately nine years.

252)   One 500-ml bottle of soda is equivalent to 10 teaspoons of sugar. To burn off these calories, an hour of exercise is necessary. To burn off a hamburger and fries, you will need to play an hour of football and a 43-minute jog.

253)   Obesity and overweight are more prevalent in countries which allow food advertising on television programmers for children and teenagers, that is one of the reasons that England has higher incidence of childhood obesity than Sweden where food advertising for children is not allowed

254)   Regarding to psychological effects of obesity in young girls and boys, women are more vulnerable than men. Low self-esteem is identified as being a very serious effect. It is more likely for young women who are obese to suffer from low self-esteem and feelings of rejection and shame than young men.

255)   Miss Ciccione d'Italia (Miss Chubby) was won this year by Angela Scognamiglio of Naples. She weighs 170 kilos (375 lbs). Her prize was an enormous cake to share with everybody. There is only one requirement to participate: You have to weigh more than 220 pounds. The organizer of the contestant, Gianfranco Lazzareschi, says it offers a new perspective on beauty. Participants say the occasion gives them a chance to regain their self-esteem.

256)   Europeans walk three times as far and cycle five times as far as Americans. In Europe, the average citizen walks an average of 240 miles each year and bike another 120. On the other hand, in the United States, Americans walk 90 miles and bike 24. This difference in exercise means that Europeans lose 8 to 10 pounds more than Americans do per year.

257)   The Swiss takes an average of 10,000 steps daily, the Japanese walks 7,500 steps every day; and in the United States, the average person takes only 6,000 steps daily. This is an important aspect when we compare the European rate of obesity against the higher rate in the United States.

258)   A study by the University of Maryland concludes that even in your elder years, a good diet is the key to obtain a longer life. Adults between seventy and eighty years old who ate more vegetables, fruits, and other healthy foods had a lower chance of death over a period of ten years than people who ate less healthy foods.

259)   In a study by the journal *Economics and Human Biology*, Oxford University researchers found that Americans and Britons are much more likely to be obese than Norwegian and Swedes. It was suggested that the stresses of life in a competitive social system, without a strong welfare state, cause people to overeat and the rate of obesity to increase. (Please change wording)

260)   Seven hundred eleven is the number of people who failed to eat. *The Belly Bruiser*, is an enormous 30,000-calorie hamburger served in a restaurant in Pennsylvania. This burger included a 22-ounce bun, 15 pounds of ground beef, and 31 pounds of cheese. Finally, Brad Sciullo won the challenge in 4 hours and 39 minutes in 2008.

261)   The annual cost to Great Britain tax payers of treatment for Paul Mason (the fattest man in England) was 100,000 pounds per year. In 2009, the year that he had a gastric surgery, the expenses were up to 1 million pounds including a specially designed, reinforced ambulance to carry him to the hospital.

262)   Of the 30 fastest growing franchises in the United States in 1999, 12 were fast-food companies.

263)   In 1999, Americans consumed an average of 55 gallons of soft drinks, 10 pounds of chocolate, and 22 pounds of chips, pretzels, and nuts per person.

In the United States, work no longer provides the opportunity for physical activity that once did., A hundred years ago in the U.S., there were 12 million farmers, now there are only 850,000. This factor increases sedentary habits and the tendency to increase weight and develop obesity.

264)   The average high school graduate in the United States will have spent approximately 15,000 to 18,000 hours in front of a television set but only about 12,000 hours in school.

265) A study conducted by researchers at John Hopkins School of Public Health found that if the trend in obesity continues at the same rate of growth, by the year 2030, 86 percent of Americans will be obese with 96 percent of non-Hispanic black women and 91 percent of Mexican American men affected. This would result in 1 of every 6 health care dollars spent in total direct health care cost paying for obesity-related costs.

266) Obese youngsters face discrimination even from their parents. In a recent study, researchers found that parents are less likely to help obese sons or daughters to pay for college. Researchers from the University of North Texas discovered also that parents are less willing to help their obese child to buy a car.

267) Wellness programs really work, companies like Johnson and Johnson claim that the *Live for Life* program saved the company $378 per employee per year by lowering absenteeism and slowing the rise in the company health-care expenses. Most of the wellness programs include exercise daily to prevent the increase of weight-related health problems.

268) General Electric, Cincinnati, found that employees that were regular exercisers were absent from work 45 percent fewer days than nonregular exercisers. The obesity-related problems are less when people exercise three to five times a week.

269) Asians have more fat content compared to Caucasians which meant that a body mass index of 25 is overweight and 30 percent is obese. Scientists are trying to figure out why Asians have more fat than Caucasians, but they believe that evolution, maternal nutrition, or simply lack of exercise are the main causes.

270) People in Asia tend to exercise less than in the West; for example, in China, less than 8 percent of China's 1.2 billion people exercise routinely. In countries like India and Malaysia, fat is a symbol of prosperity.

271) The risk of developing diabetes increase with overweight and obesity. In the United States, the Centers for Disease

Control (CDC) estimate the number of diabetic Americans in 26 millions. This marks a 9-percent increase from the 2008 estimates of 23.6 million and means that 1 in every 12 Americans is diabetic.

272) "A team of researchers led by Tim Key of Oxford University has found that meat eaters who switched a plant-based diet gained less weight over a period of five years, as well as a study of more than 55,000 Swedish women showing that meat eaters are more likely to be overweight as vegetarians."

273) *Women En Large*, a book by Debbie Notkin, has sold over 9,000 copies around the world. It is used as a textbook in gender studies and portrays obese nude women.

274) In some cultures, obesity is associated with strength and fertility; in cultures prone to food scarcity, obesity functions as a symbol of success and wealth.

275) Obesity in French women and men climbed from approximately 8 percent in 1998 to 11 percent in 2003, an increase of almost 40 percent.

276) The State of California alone spends $22 billion in obesity-related expenses per year.

277) A recent report has revealed that the number of children being prescribed diet medicines like Reductil and Xenical has dramatically increased over the last decade. Since the year 2000, the number of prescriptions written for teenagers has climbed 15 fold.

278) An increased number of obese school children are suffering from back pain as consequence of the small size of school furniture. Replacing the furniture is really important to prevent having back problems.

279) Scientists estimated that the solid fats found in margarine, cakes, and junk foods were responsible for a significant number of deaths every year. Some groups are trying to ban completely this type of fats.

280) Seaweed could be a powerful treatment to fight obesity. Scientists have determined that the fiber found in sea kelp can reduce the update of fat by the body by up to 75 percent,

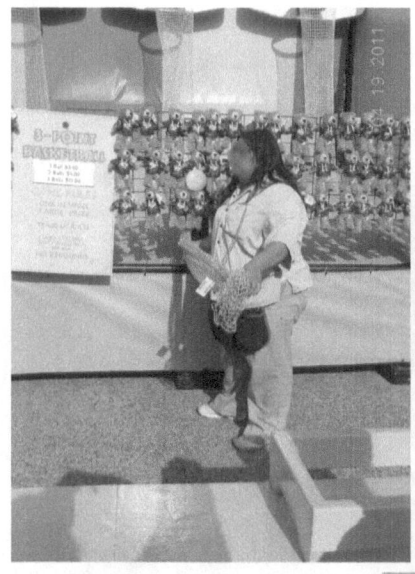

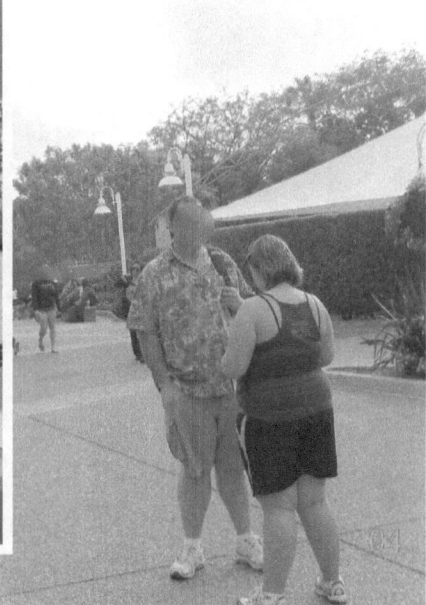

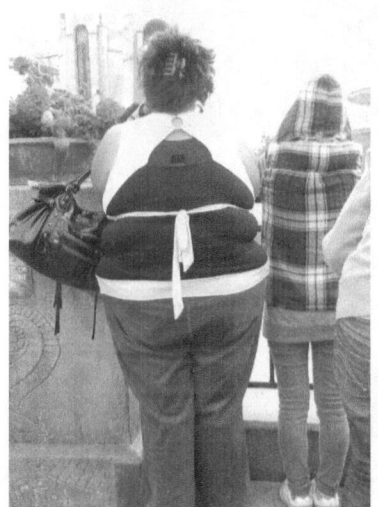

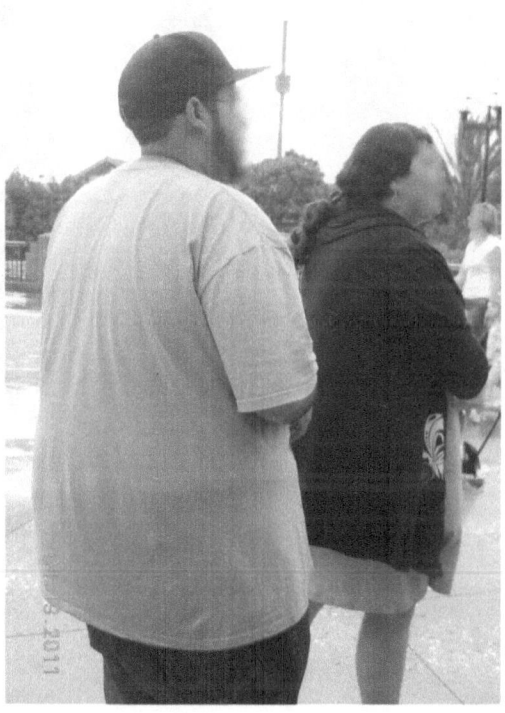

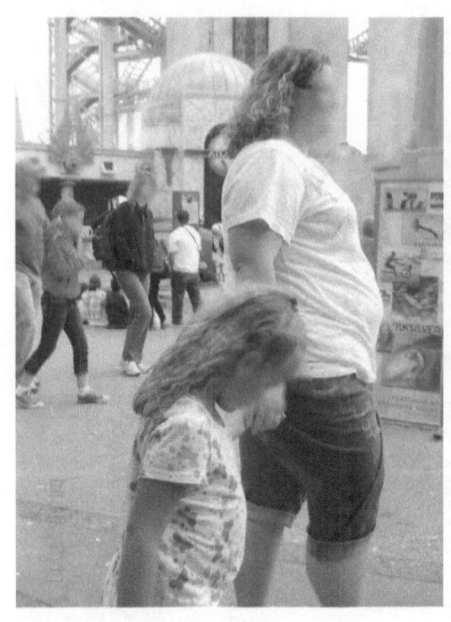

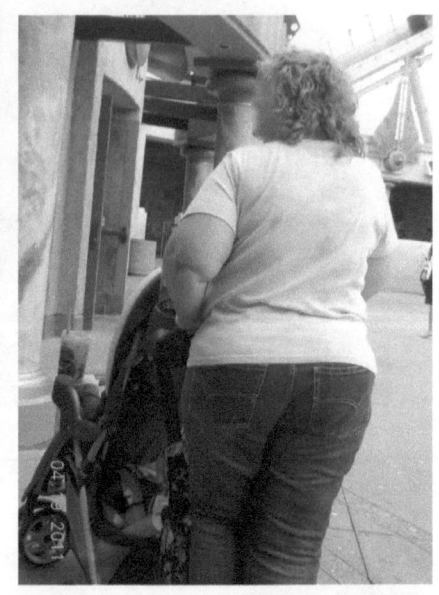

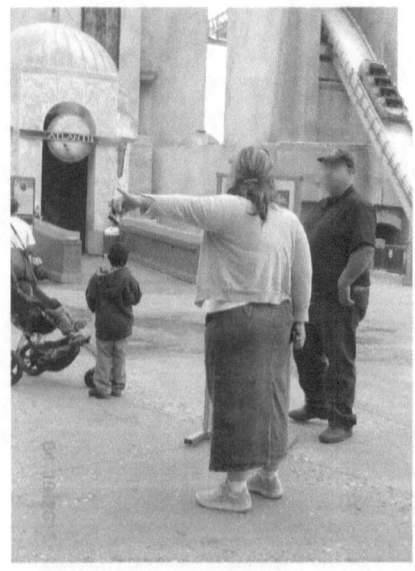

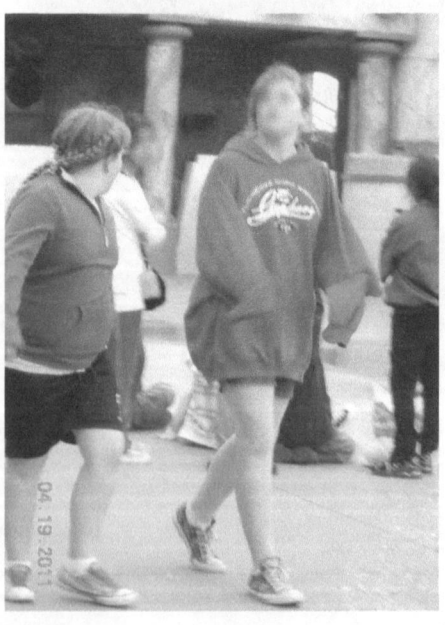

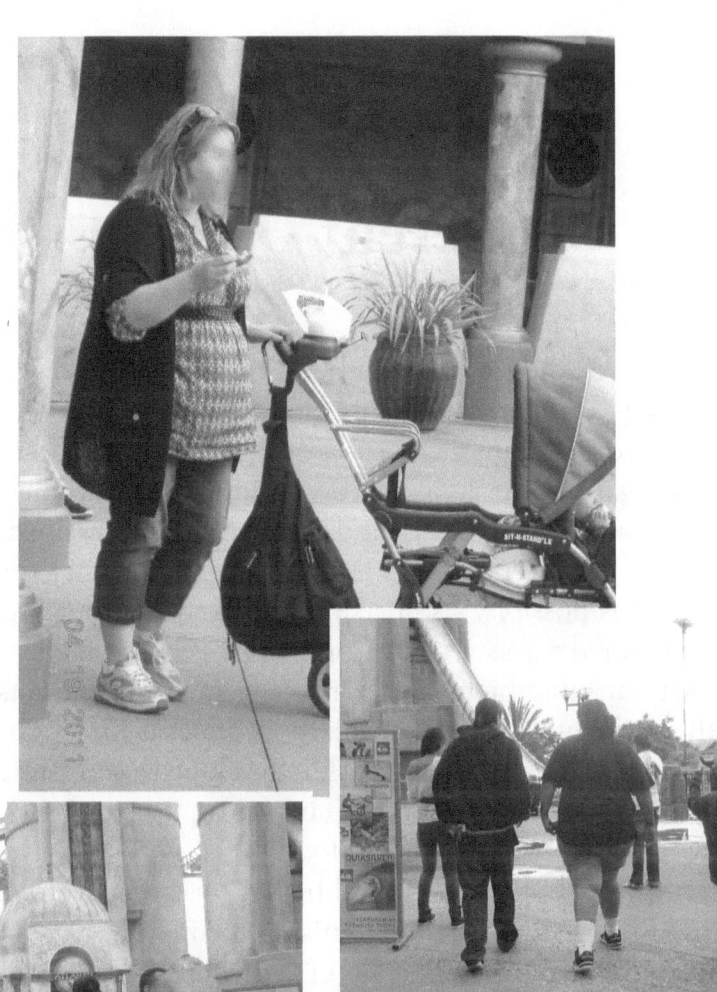

CHAPTER 5

Different Diets

281) The word "diet" comes from Old French *diete* and Medieval Latin *dieta* that means "daily food allowance."

282) Atkins diet: Atkins diet focuses on controlling insulin levels in our organism through diet. Every time we eat carbohydrates, our insulin levels rise fast and then fall sharply. Rising insulin levels will trigger our organism to store as much of the energy we eat as possible, also make it less likely that our organism uses stored fat as a source of energy. People on the Atkins Diet consume higher proportion of proteins and fats than they normally do. Intake of carbohydrates is limited because for four and half million years, it developed a gastrointestinal system that was based on proteins (meat, fish, and fowl) men. Women were recollectors of food.

283) South Beach diet was started by Dr. Agatson, a cardiologist, and Marie Almon, a nutritionist. It focuses on the control of insulin levels and the benefits of slow carbohydrates compared to fast carbohydrates. Dr. Agatson found out that low-fat diets are not effective over the long term. South Beach diet was first used during the 1990s.

284) Vegan diet: Veganism is more a way of life than a diet, a vegan does not eat anything that is animal based. This includes honey, eggs, and dairy products.

285) Raw Food diet: This way of eating involves consuming food which is not processed and is completely plant based, and preference is given to organic foods. For raw food eaters, 75 percent of their food intake should be uncooked food. There

are four main types of raw foods; (a) raw vegetarians, (b) raw carnivores (raw meat, for example, sushi), (c) raw omnivores (eat raw vegetables and raw meat), and (d) raw vegans.

286) Mediterranean diet: This diet comes from Southern Europe: Spain, Greece, Italy. The emphasis is on lots of fruits, nuts, plant foods, olive oil, cheese and yogurt, fish and poultry. It limits the number of eggs to a maximum of five per week, moderate amount of wine and moderate red meat. Thirty percent of the Mediterranean diet consists of fats with saturated fats not exceeding 8 percent of the total calorie intake.

287) The Zone diet: The diet goal is a nutritional balance of 40 percent carbohydrates, 30 percent fats, and 30 percent protein every time we eat. The Zone diet encourages the intake of good-quality carbohydrates (unrefined carbohydrates and fats, such as olive oil, avocado, and nuts).

288) Vegetarian diet: The majority of vegetarians are lacto-ovo vegetarians; they do not eat animal-based foods except for eggs, honey, and dairy products. Recent studies have shown that vegetarians have a lower body weight and generally have a longer life expectancy than people who eat meat.

289) Weight Watchers diet: This focuses on losing weight through exercise, diet, and support group. Weight Watchers Incorporated was born in 1960s. Weight Watchers is a large company with branches all over the world.

Fruit Diet:

This is a diet based on wonder fruits.

290) Grapefruit: Pulp of this fruit reduces cancer including precancerous conditions in smokers and other people and lowers bad cholesterol up to 20 percent because of the great amount of antioxidants

291) Coconut: It is considered a super fruit, the best thing that you can eat. The people, especially in Asia, that eat coconut

avoid cardiovascular diseases and cancer. The coconut oil avoids heart disease, atherosclerosis, colon cancer, and digestive problems. Half of a cup of coconut meat contains approximately 142 milligrams of potassium, almost 5 grams of fiber and 14 grams of heart-healthy nutrients. The fattening acids from the coconut work against diarrhea. The coconut is antiviral, so it helps against antibacterial like herpes, chlamydia, and other venereal diseases.

292)   Cherries: They act as anti-inflammatory, antiaging, and fight allergies and asthma. They also reduce colon cancer and gout pain.

293)   Cantaloupe: the best friend of weight control. One cup of melon cubes contains potassium, calcium, and magnesium which are aids of a healthy blood pressure. Five cups of cantaloupe daily decrease blood pressure up 20 percent. Cantaloupe is rich in vitamin A. If you don't have it, your resistance to infection and your immune system goes down up to 25 percent.

294)   Blueberries: They are antioxidants and anti-inflammatory and help Parkinson's disease, diabetes, and heart disease. Blueberry keeps your memory sharp at all times and attacks cardiovascular disease.

295)   Banana: Between 4 and 5 grams of fiber per banana, it helps to maintain cell integrity and keeps heart rate steady and is excellent in controlling hypertension. And if you don't eat bananas, your risk of kidney cancer doubles.

296)   Avocado: It helps to decrease cholesterol. It's great for your skin, your heart, and your eyes, just by eating a small avocado a day.

297)   Apricots: They tend to reduce the risk of lung and colon cancer. They reduce lung cancer for more than 35 percent and arthritis by 40 percent.

298)   Peaches: They have low calories, one and half grams of fiber, vitamin C, vitamin K, and have significant amounts of magnesium, phosphorus, and calcium. The carotenoids in the peach are anti-inflammatory and anticancer. The

peach is a super star fruit because of its great antimicrobial, antioxidant activity, and tumor growth inhibition.

299)   Papaya: Legend says that papaya was named as the "fruit of the angels" by Christopher Columbus. It is considered one of the best, to say the least, to protect the digestive tract. Thanks to the enzyme papain. Papaya is a heavyweight in potassium, so it reduces approximately 30 percent the risk of lung cancer.

300)   Orange: Two glasses of natural orange juice daily decrease chances of stroke by 30 percent. Vitamin C is one of the best antioxidants on earth, helping all the cells. Together with the antioxidants, it reduces high blood pressure, inflammation, and bad cholesterol; and on top, it contains calcium that keeps teeth and bones healthy.

301)   Mango: This fruit has a lot of potassium, beta-carotene, vitamin C, calcium, phosphorus, magnesium, and other nutrients. Mango is rich in enzymes, one mango (average size) contains 4 grams of fiber, and mango is another wonder fruit.

302)   Kiwi: It contains double amount of vitamin C than oranges. The index of nutrition of kiwi is 16, definitely the densest of all fruits. For you to have an idea, the second place is papaya with 14, and the third is a tie between mango and orange with an index of 11. It thins the blood naturally without aspirin.

303)   Guava: It is considered among the ten top fruits. It contains antioxidants that protect all the cells including the DNA. Guava can help prevent cancer.

304)   Fig: Fig is the equivalent of fiber. You should eat between 30 and 50 grams of figs a day. If you don't, you have 40 percent more probabilities of heart attack

305)   Fad dieting appears first in 1829. Sylvester Graham, a Presbyterian minister, developed a diet based on caffeine-free drinks, vegetarian food, and graham crackers as cure, not only for obesity, but for masturbation (Graham Diet).

306)   In 1857, Dr. Gustav Zander of Sweden invented the first belt-driven fat massager.

307)   In 1864, William Banting in England became famous by using a low carbohydrate diet which helped him lose 23 kilograms. The same year, he published the book *Letter on Corpulence*. This diet became so popular that "banting" became a synonym for dieting. Early editions sold sixty thousand copies of the book.

308)   In 1903, Horace Fletcher became known as the "Great Masticator" and developed the idea that one should chew food exactly thirty-two times before spitting out. (No swallowing was allowed.) Fletcher claimed to lose 60 pounds by using this technique.

309)   In 1917, Lulu Hunt Peters wrote the book *Diet in Health with the Key to the Calories*. The Peter's system was based in calorie counting and promoted 1,200 calories a day. He sold two million copies of his book.

310)   In 1925, the Cigarette diet was developed to promote smoking instead of eating sweets. This diet was based on the appetite-suppressing properties of tobacco.

311)   In 1995, supposedly a tablet existed to allow to swallow a parasite, this was known as the Tapeworm Diet. According to legend, the obese singer Maria Callas lost 70 pounds with the help of this diet.

312)   Other fad diets are the Scarsdale Diet, the Cabbage Diet, the Astronaut's Diet, the Sleeping Beauty Diet, the Blood Type Diet, the F Diet, the Hay Diet, and many more.

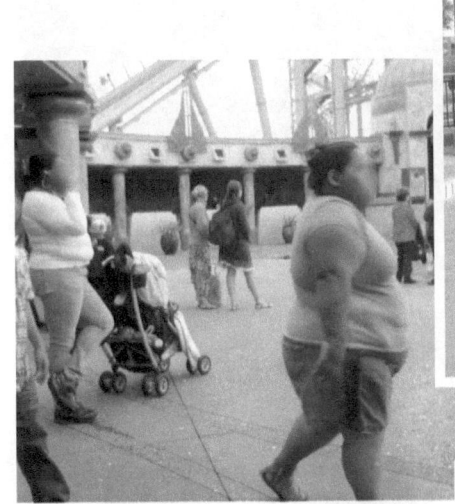
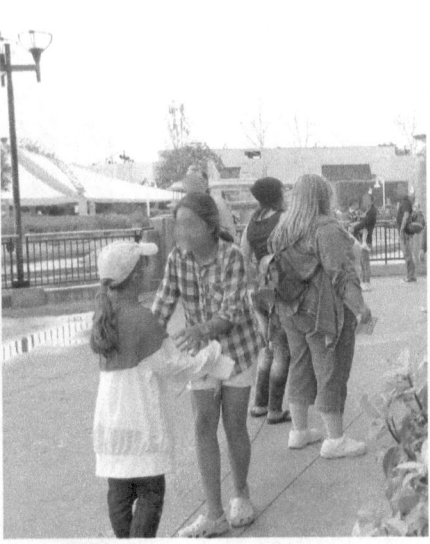
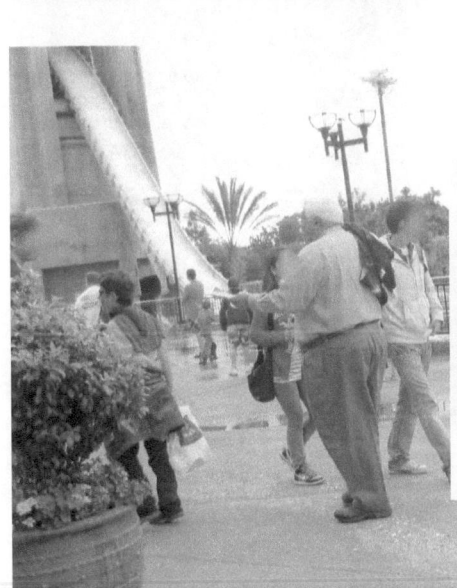
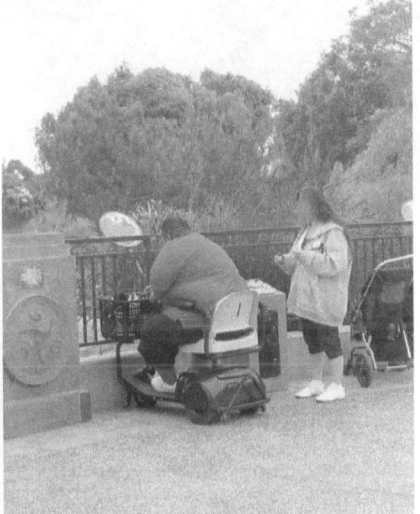

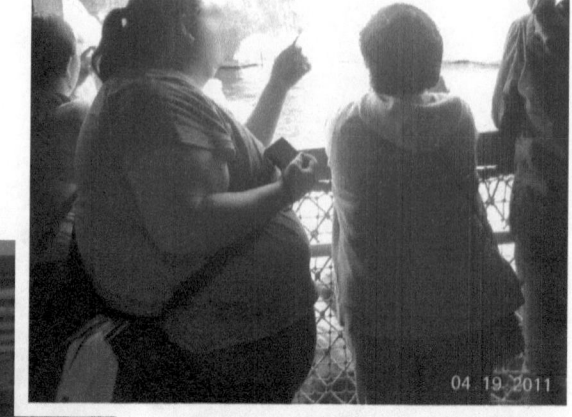

04.19.2011

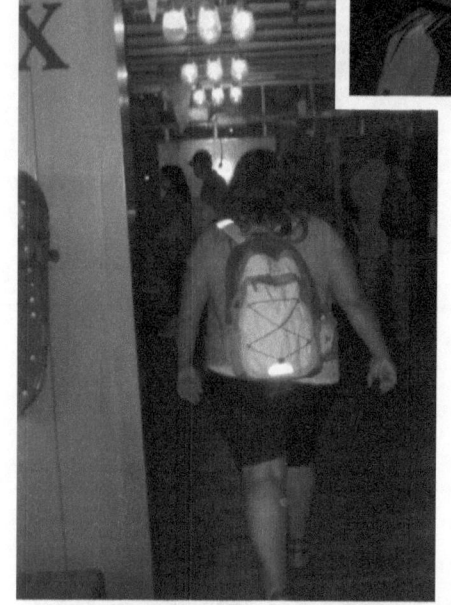

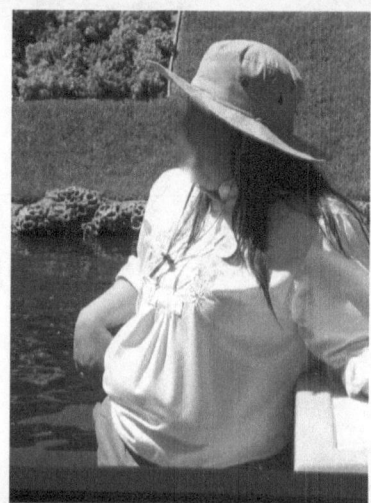

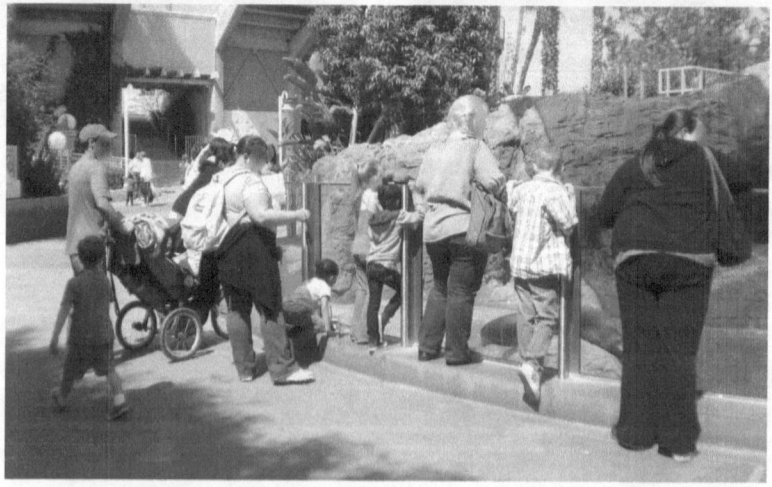

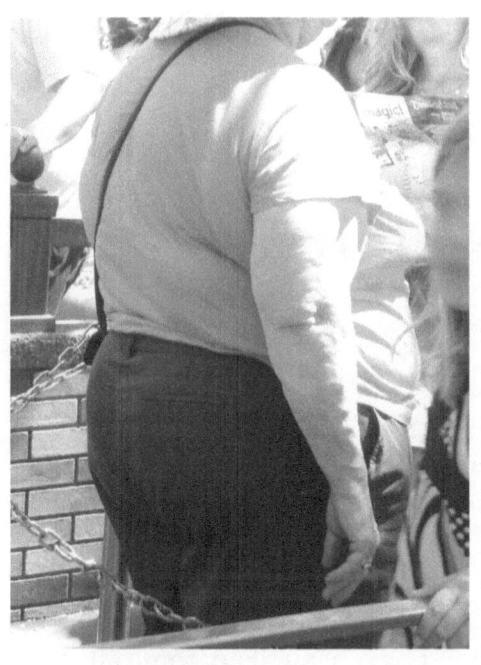

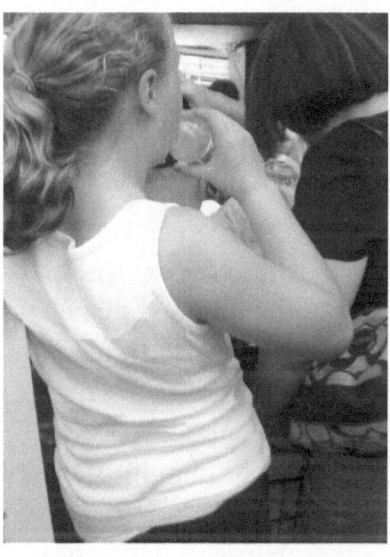

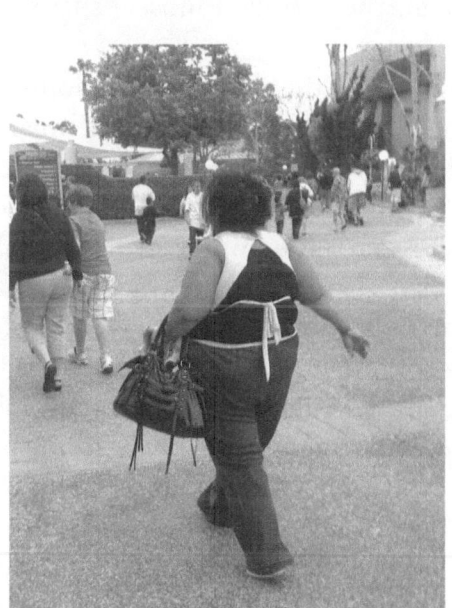

CHAPTER 6

Glossary of Terms

313) **Abdomen:** The belly, that part of the body that contains all of the structures between the chest and the pelvis. The abdomen is separated anatomically from the chest by the diaphragm, the powerful muscle spanning the body cavity below the lungs.

314) **Abdominal:** Relating to the abdomen, the belly, that part of the body that contains all of the structures between the chest and the pelvis. The abdomen is separated anatomically from the chest by the diaphragm, the powerful muscle spanning the body cavity below the lungs.

315) **Abdominal pain:** Pain in the belly (the abdomen). Abdominal pain can come from conditions affecting a variety of organs. The abdomen is an anatomical area that is bounded by the lower margin of the ribs above, the pelvic bone (*pubic ramus*) below, and the flanks on each side. Although abdominal pain can arise from the tissues of the abdominal wall that surround the abdominal cavity (the skin and abdominal wall muscles), the term abdominal pain is generally used to describe pain originating from organs within the abdominal cavity (from beneath the skin and muscles). These organs include the stomach, small intestine, colon, liver, gallbladder, and pancreas.

316) **Abnormal:** Not normal. Deviating from the usual structure, position, condition, or behavior. In referring to a growth, abnormal may mean that it is cancerous or premalignant (likely to become *cancer*).

317) **Absorption:** Uptake. In the biomedical sciences, absorption has diverse specific meanings.

318) **Amino acid:** One of the 20 building blocks of protein. The sequence of amino acids in a protein and, hence, the function of that protein are determined by the genetic code in the DNA.

319) **Analysis:** A psychology term for processes used to gain understanding of complex emotional or behavioral issues.

320) **Anemia:** The condition of having less than the normal number of red blood cells or less than the normal quantity of hemoglobin in the blood. The oxygen-carrying capacity of the blood is, therefore, decreased.

321) **Anesthesia:** Loss of feeling or awareness. A general *anesthetic* puts the person to *sleep*. A local anesthetic causes loss of feeling in a part of the body such as a tooth or an area of skin without affecting consciousness. Regional anesthesia numbs a larger part of the body such as a leg or arm, also without affecting consciousness. The term "conduction anesthesia" encompasses both local and regional anesthetic techniques. Many surgical procedures can be done with conduction anesthesia without significant *pain*. In many situations, such as a *C-section*, conduction anesthesia is safer and therefore preferable to general anesthesia. However, there are also many types of surgery in which general anesthesia is clearly appropriate.

322) **Ankle:** The ankle joint is complex. It is made up of two joints; the true ankle joint and the subtalar joint.

323) **Antidepressants:** Anything, and especially a drug, used to prevent or treat depression.

324) **Antihistamines:** Drugs that combat the histamine released during an allergic reaction by blocking the action of the histamine on the tissue. Antihistamines do not stop the formation of histamine nor do they stop the conflict between the IgE and antigen. Therefore, antihistamines do not stop the allergic reaction but protect tissues from some of its effects. Antihistamines frequently cause mouth dryness and sleepiness. Newer nonsedating antihistamines are generally

thought to be somewhat less effective. Antihistamine side effects that very occasionally occur include urine retention in males and fast heart rate.

325) **Apnea:** An apnea is a period of time during which breathing stops or is markedly reduced. There are two types of apneas, the more common is obstructive sleep apnea, and the less common is central sleep apnea.

326) **Artery:** A vessel that carries blood high in oxygen content away from the heart to the farthest reaches of the body. Since blood in arteries is usually full of oxygen, the hemoglobin in the red blood cells is oxygenated. The resultant form of hemoglobin (oxyhemoglobin) is what makes arterial blood look bright red.

327) **Arthritis:** Inflammation of a joint. When joints are inflamed, they can develop stiffness, warmth, swelling, redness, and pain. There are over one hundred types of *arthritis*.

328) *http://www.medicinenet.com/obesity_weight_loss/glossary.htm–backtotop*
Aspartame: A man-made sweetener with almost no calories used in place of sugar.

329) **Asthma:** A common disorder in which chronic inflammation of the bronchial tubes (bronchi) makes them swell, narrowing the airways. Asthma involves only the bronchial tubes and does not affect the air sacs (alveoli) or the lung tissue (the parenchyma of the lung) itself.

330) **Atherosclerosis:** A process of progressive thickening and hardening of the walls of medium-sized and large arteries as a result of fat deposits on their inner lining.

331) **Bariatric:** Pertaining to *bariatrics*, the field of medicine concerned with weight loss.

332) **Bariatric surgery:** Surgery on the stomach and/or intestines to help a person with extreme obesity lose weight. Bariatric surgery is an option for people who have a body mass index (BMI) above 40. Surgery is also an option for people with a BMI between 35 and 40 who have health problems like type 2 diabetes or heart disease.

333) **Baseline: 1.** Information gathered at the beginning of a study from which variations found in the study are measured.

2. A known value or quantity with which an unknown is compared when measured or assessed.

3. The initial time point in a clinical trial, just before a participant starts to receive the experimental treatment which is being tested. At this reference point, measurable values such as CD4 count are recorded. Safety and efficacy of a drug are often determined by monitoring changes from the baseline values.

334) **Belly:** That part of the body that contains all of the structures between the chest and the pelvis. Also called the abdomen.

335) **Bioelectric impedance analysis:** A seemingly simple method for determining the *lean body mass*. Abbreviated as BIA. There are two methods of the BIA. One involves standing on a special scale with footpads. A harmless amount of electrical current is sent through the body, and then the percentage of body fat is calculated. The other type of BIA involves electrodes usually placed on a wrist and an ankle and on the back of the right hand and on the top of the foot. The change in voltage between electrodes is measured. The person's body fat percentage is then calculated from the results of the BIA.

336) **Blood clots:** Blood that has been converted from a liquid to a solid state. Also called a thrombus.

337) **Blood glucose:** The main sugar that the body makes from the food in the diet. Glucose is carried through the bloodstream to provide energy to all cells in the body. Cells cannot use glucose without the help of insulin.

338) **Blood pressure:** The blood pressure is the pressure of the *blood* within the arteries. It is produced primarily by the *contraction* of the *heart muscle*. Its measurement is recorded by two numbers. The first (*systolic* pressure) is measured after the *heart* contracts and is highest. The second (*diastolic* pressure) is measured before the heart contracts and lowest. A blood pressure cuff is used to measure the pressure. Elevation of blood pressure is called *hypertension*.

339) **Blood sugar:** *Blood glucose.* See also *High blood sugar; Low blood sugar.*

340) **BMI:** *Body mass index.*

341) **BOD POD:** A method for determining the *lean body mass.* The BOD POD is a computerized, egg-shaped chamber. Using the same whole-body measurement principle as *underwater weighing,* the BOD POD measures a subject's mass and volume, from which their whole-body density is determined. Using these data, body fat and lean muscle mass can then be calculated.

342) **Body mass index:** A key index for relating a person's body weight to their height. The body mass index (BMI) is a person's weight in kilograms (kg) divided by their height in meters (m) squared.

343) **Bone density:** Bone density is the amount of bone tissue in a certain volume of bone. It can be measured using a special x-ray called a quantitative computed tomogram.

344) **Bowel:** Another name for the intestine. The small bowel and the large bowel are the small intestine and large intestine, respectively.

345) **Brain:** That part of the *central nervous system* that is located within the *cranium (skull).* The brain functions as the primary receiver, organizer and distributor of information for the body. It has two (right and left) halves called "hemispheres."

346) **Breast cancer:** *Breast cancer* is diagnosed with self—and physician-examination of the breasts, mammography, ultrasound testing, and biopsy. There are many types of breast cancer that differ in their capability of spreading to other body tissues (metastasis). Treatment of breast cancer depends on the type and location of the breast cancer, as well as the age and health of the patient. The American Cancer Society recommends that a woman should have a baseline mammogram between the ages of thirty-five and forty years. Between forty and fifty years of age mammograms are recommended every other year. After age fifty years, yearly mammograms are recommended.

347) **Bypass:** An operation in which a surgeon creates a new tubular pathway for the movement of fluids and/or other substances in the body.

348) **Caffeine:** A stimulant found naturally in coffee beans, tea leaves, cocoa beans (chocolate) and kola nuts (cola) and added to soft drinks, foods, and medicines. A cup of coffee has 100–250 milligrams of caffeine. Black tea brewed for 4 minutes has 40–100 milligrams. Green tea has one-third as much caffeine as black tea.

349) **Calipers:** A metal or plastic tool similar to a compass used to measure the diameter of an object. The skin fold thickness in several parts of the body can be measured with *skin calipers* to determine the *lean body mass*. This may be done in medicine, physical anthropology, health clubs, and athletic facilities.

350) **Calorie:** A unit of food energy. In *nutrition* terms, the word calorie is used instead of the more precise scientific term kilocalorie which represents the amount of energy required to raise the temperature of a liter of water one degree centigrade at sea level. The common usage of the word calorie of food energy is understood to refer to a kilocalorie and actually represents, therefore, 1000 true calories of energy. A calorie is also known as cal, gram calorie, or small calorie.

351) **Cancer:** An abnormal growth of cells which tend to proliferate in an uncontrolled way and, in some cases, to metastasize (spread).

352) **Carbohydrates:** Mainly sugars and starches, together constituting one of the three principal types of nutrients used as energy sources (calories) by the body. Carbohydrates can also be defined chemically as neutral compounds of carbon, hydrogen and oxygen.

353) **Cerebrovascular:** Pertaining to the blood vessels and, especially, the arteries that supply the brain. As in cerebrovascular accident or cerebrovascular disease.

354) **Cerebrovascular accident:** The sudden death of some brain cells due to lack of oxygen when the blood flow to the brain is impaired by blockage or rupture of an artery to the brain. A CVA is also referred to as a stroke.

355) **Chest:** The area of the body located between the neck and the abdomen. The chest contains the lungs, the heart and

part of the aorta. The walls of the chest are supported by the dorsal vertebrae, the ribs, and the sternum.

356) **Cholesterol:** The most common type of steroid in the body, cholesterol has gotten something of a bad name. However, cholesterol is a critically important molecule.

357) **Chronic:** This important term in medicine comes from the Greek chronos, time and means lasting a long time.

358) **Chronic disease:** A disease that persists for a long time. A chronic disease is one lasting three months or more, by the definition of the U.S. National Center for Health Statistics. Chronic diseases generally cannot be prevented by vaccines or cured by medication, nor do they just disappear. Eighty-eight percent of Americans over sixty-five years of age have at least one chronic health condition (as of 1998). Health damaging behaviors—particularly tobacco use, lack of physical activity, and poor eating habits—are major contributors to the leading chronic diseases.

359) **Clinical trials:** Trials to evaluate the effectiveness and safety of medications or medical devices by monitoring their effects on large groups of people.

360) **Colon:** The part of the large intestine that runs from the cecum to the rectum as a long hollow tube that serves to remove water from digested food and let the remaining material, solid waste called stool, move through it to the rectum and leave the body through the anus. .

361) **Congestive heart failure:** Inability of the heart to keep up with the demands on it and, specifically, failure of the heart to pump blood with normal efficiency. When this occurs, the heart is unable to provide adequate blood flow to other organs such as the brain, liver and kidneys. Heart failure may be due to failure of the right or left or both ventricles. The signs and symptoms depend upon which side of the heart is failing. They can include shortness of breath (dyspnea), asthma due to the heart (cardiac asthma), pooling of blood (stasis) in the general body (systemic) circulation or in the liver's (portal) circulation, swelling (edema), blueness or duskiness (cyanosis), and enlargement (hypertrophy) of the heart.

362) **Coronary artery disease:** A major cause of illness and death, coronary artery disease (CAD) begins when hard cholesterol substances (plaques) are deposited within a coronary artery.

363) **Deep vein thrombosis:** A blood clot (thrombus) in a deep vein in the thigh or leg. The clot can break off as an embolus and make its way to the lung, where it can cause respiratory distress and respiratory failure.

364) **Degenerative arthritis:** Also known as *osteoarthritis*, this type of *arthritis* is caused by inflammation, breakdown and eventual loss of the cartilage of the joints. Among the over 100 different types of arthritis conditions, osteoarthritis is the most common, affecting usually the hands, feet, spine, and large weight-bearing joints, such as the hips and knees. Also called degenerative joint disease.

365) **Dehydration:** Excessive loss of body water. Diseases of the gastrointestinal tract that cause vomiting or diarrhea and may, for example, lead to dehydration. There are a number of other causes of dehydration including heat exposure, prolonged vigorous exercise (e.g., in a marathon), kidney disease, and medications (diuretics).

366) **Depression:** An illness that involves the body, mood, and thoughts, that affects the way a person eats and sleeps, the way one feels about oneself, and the way one thinks about things. A depressive disorder is not the same as a passing blue mood. It is not a sign of personal weakness or a condition that can be wished away. People with a depressive disease cannot merely "pull themselves together" and get better. Without treatment, symptoms can last for weeks, months, or years. Appropriate treatment, however, can help most people with depression.

367) **DEXA:** Dual-energy x-ray absorptometry.

368) **Dexfenfluramine:** A weight loss drug, in a class of drugs called anorectics which decrease appetite. This drug, sold in the US under the brand name Redux, was withdrawn from the US market in 1997, and has since been withdrawn worldwide and is no longer available because of its association with abnormal heart valve findings, primarily aortic regurgitation.

369) **Diabetes:** Refers to diabetes mellitus or, less often, to diabetes insipidus. Diabetes mellitus and diabetes insipidus share the name "diabetes" because they are both conditions characterized by excessive urination (polyuria).

370) *http://www.medicinenet.com/obesity_weight_loss/glossary.htm–backtotop* **Diarrhea:** A familiar phenomenon with unusually frequent or unusually liquid bowel movements, excessive watery evacuations of fecal material. It is the opposite of constipation. The word "diarrhea" with its odd spelling is a near-steal from the Greek *diarrhoia*, meaning "a flowing through." Plato and Aristotle may have had *diarrhoia* while today we have diarrhea. There are myriad infectious and noninfectious causes of diarrhea.

371) **Discharge:** 1. The flow of fluid from part of the body, such as from the nose or vagina.

    2. The passing of an action potential, such as through a nerve or muscle *fiber*.

    3. The release of a patient from a course of care. The doctor may then dictate a discharge summary.

372) **Dopamine:** An important neurotransmitter (messenger) in the brain.

373) **Embolism:** The obstruction of a blood vessel by a foreign substance or a blood clot blocking the vessel. Something travels through the bloodstream, lodges in a vessel, and plugs it.

374) **Enzymes:** Proteins that act as a catalyst in mediating and speeding a specific chemical reaction.

375) **Epidemic:** The occurrence of more cases of a disease than would be expected in a community or region during a given time period. A sudden severe outbreak of a disease such as SARS. From the Greek *epi*–which means "upon" and *demos*, which means "people or population." *Epidemos* means "upon the population." See also Endemic; Pandemic.

376) **Esophagus:** The tube that connects the pharynx (throat) with the stomach. The esophagus lies between the trachea (windpipe) and the spine. It passes down the neck, pierces the diaphragm just to the left of the midline, and joins the

cardiac (upper) end of the stomach. In an adult, the esophagus is about 25 centimeters (10 inches) long. When a person swallows, the muscular walls of the esophagus contract to push food down into the stomach. Glands in the lining of the esophagus produce mucus which keeps the passageway moist and facilitates swallowing. It is also known as the gullet or swallowing tube. From the Greek *oisophagos*, from oisein meaning to bear or carry, and *phagein*, to eat.

377) **Essential: 1.** Something that cannot be done without.

    2. Required in the diet because the body cannot make it, as in an essential amino acid or an essential fatty acid.

    3. Idiopathic. As in essential hypertension. "Essential" is a hallowed term meaning "We don't know the cause."

378) **Estrogen:** Estrogen is a female hormone produced by the ovaries. Estrogen deficiency can lead to osteoporosis.

379) **Fatigue:** A condition characterized by a lessened capacity for work and reduced efficiency of accomplishment, usually accompanied by a feeling of weariness and tiredness. Fatigue can be acute or chronic and comes on suddenly and persist.

380) **Fats:** Plural of the word "fat." See the definition of *fat*.

381) **FDA:** The Food and Drug Administration, an agency within the U.S. Public Health Service, which is a part of the Department of Health and Human Services.

382) **Fenfluramine:** A *weight loss* drug, in a class of drugs called anorectics which decrease appetite. This drug, sold in the U.S. under the brand name *Pondimin*, was withdrawn from the U.S. market in 1997 and has since been withdrawn worldwide and is no longer available because of its association with abnormal heart valve findings, primarily *aortic regurgitation*.

383) **Food and Drug Administration:** The FDA, an agency within the U.S. Public Health Service, which is a part of the Department of Health and Human Services.

384) **Forceps:** An instrument with two blades and a handle used for handling, grasping, or compressing. Many types of forceps are employed in medicine, including the alligator forceps (an angled instrument with jaws at the end), tissue forceps

(a form of tweezer), hemostatic forceps (also simply called a hemostat, to clamp a bleeding vessel), mosquito forceps (a small hemostat), and obstetrical forceps (to aid in delivering a baby).

385)   *http://www.medicinenet.com/obesity_weight_loss/glossary.htm–backtotop*
        Fructose: A sugar that occurs naturally in fruits and honey. Fructose has 4 calories per gram.

386)   **Gallbladder:** A pear-shaped organ just below the liver that stores the bile secreted by the liver. During a fatty meal, the gallbladder contracts, delivering the bile through the bile ducts into the intestines to help with digestion. Abnormal composition of bile leads to formation of *gallstones*, a process termed *cholelithiasis*. The gallstones cause *cholecystitis*, an inflammation of the gallbladder.

387)   **Gallstones:** Stones that form when substances in the bile harden. Gallstones can be as small as a grain of sand or as large as a golf ball. There can be just one large stone, hundreds of tiny stones, or any combination.

388)   **Gastric:** Having to do with the stomach.

389)   **Gastric banding:** A surgically implanted device used to help a person lose weight. In a surgical procedure, a band is placed around the upper part of the stomach, creating a small pouch that can hold only a small amount of food. The narrowed opening between the stomach pouch and the rest of the stomach controls how quickly food passes from the pouch to the lower part of the stomach. The system helps the patient eat less by limiting the amount of food that can be eaten at one time and increasing the time it takes for food to be digested.

390)   **Gastrointestinal:** Adjective referring collectively to the stomach and small and large intestines.

391)   **Gastrointestinal tract:** The tube that extends from the mouth to the anus in which the movement of muscles and release of hormones and enzymes digest food. The gastrointestinal tract starts with the mouth and proceeds to the esophagus, stomach, duodenum, small intestine, large

intestine (colon), rectum, and, finally, the anus. Also called the alimentary canal, digestive tract, and, perhaps most often in conversation, the GI tract.

392) **Genetic:** Having to do with genes and genetic information.

393) **Genetic disease:** A disease caused by an abnormality in an individual's genome.

394) **Genetics:** The scientific study of heredity. Genetics pertains to humans and all other organisms. So, for example, there is human genetics, mouse genetics, fruit genetics, etc.

395) **Glucose:** The simple sugar (monosaccharide) that serves as the chief source of energy in the body. Glucose is the principal sugar the body makes. The body makes glucose from proteins, fats, and, in largest part, carbohydrates. Glucose is carried to each cell through the bloodstream. Cells, however, cannot use glucose without the help of insulin. Glucose is also known as dextrose.

396) **Gout:** Condition characterized by abnormally elevated levels of uric acid in the blood, recurring attacks of joint inflammation (*arthritis*), deposits of hard lumps of uric acid in and around the joints, and decreased kidney function and *kidney stones*. Uric acid is a breakdown product of purines that are part of many foods we eat. The tendency to develop *gout* and elevated blood uric acid level (hyperuricemia) is often inherited and can be promoted by *obesity*, weight gain, alcohol intake, *high blood pressure*, abnormal kidney function, and drugs. The most reliable diagnostic test for gout is the identification of crystals in joints, body fluids, and tissues.

397) **HDL:** High density lipoprotein.

398) **HDL cholesterol:** Lipoproteins, which are combinations of lipids (fats) and proteins, are the form in which lipids are transported in the blood. The high-density lipoproteins transport cholesterol from the tissues of the body to the liver so it can be gotten rid of (in the bile). HDL cholesterol is therefore considered the "good" cholesterol. The higher the HDL cholesterol level, the lower the risk of coronary artery disease.

399)   **Headache:** A pain in the head with the pain being above the eyes or the ears, behind the head (occipital), or in the back of the upper neck. Headache, like chest pain or backache, has many causes.

400)   *http://www.medicinenet.com/obesity_weight_loss/glossary.htm—backtotop*
Health for All: A global health movement undertaken by the World Health Organization (WHO) in the late twentieth century.

401)   **Heart:** The muscle that pumps blood received from veins into arteries throughout the body. It is positioned in the chest behind the sternum (breastbone; in front of the trachea, esophagus, and aorta; and above the diaphragm muscle that separates the chest and abdominal cavities). The normal heart is about the size of a closed fist and weighs about 10.5 ounces. It is cone-shaped, with the point of the cone pointing down to the left. Two-thirds of the heart lies in the left side of the chest with the balance in the right chest.

402)   **Heart attack:** The death of heart muscle due to the loss of blood supply. The loss of blood supply is usually caused by a complete blockage of a coronary artery, one of the arteries that supplies blood to the heart muscle. Death of the heart muscle, in turn, causes chest pain and electrical instability of the heart muscle tissue.

403)   **Heart disease:** Any disorder that affects the heart. Sometimes the term "heart disease" is used narrowly and incorrectly as a synonym for *coronary artery disease*. *Heart disease* is synonymous with cardiac disease but not with cardiovascular disease, which is any disease of the heart or blood vessels. Examples of the many types of heart disease are the following: angina, arrhythmia, congenital heart disease, coronary artery disease (CAD), dilated cardiomyopathy, heart attack (myocardial infarction), heart failure, hypertrophic cardiomyopathy, mitral regurgitation, mitral valve prolapse, and pulmonary stenosis.

404)   **Heart failure:** Inability of the heart to keep up with the demands on it and, specifically, failure of the heart to pump

blood with normal efficiency. When this occurs, the heart is unable to provide adequate blood flow to other organs such as the brain, liver, and kidneys. Heart failure may be due to failure of the right or left or both ventricles. The signs and symptoms depend upon which side of the heart is failing. They can include shortness of breath (dyspnea), asthma due to the heart (cardiac asthma), pooling of blood (stasis) in the general body (systemic) circulation or in the liver's (portal) circulation, swelling (edema), blueness or duskiness (cyanosis), and enlargement (hypertrophy) of the heart.

405)   **Heart valves:** There are four heart valves. All are one-way valves. Blood entering the heart first passes through the tricuspid valve and then the pulmonary valve. After returning from the lungs, the blood passes through the mitral (bicuspid) valve and exits via the aortic valve.

406)   **Herbal: 1.** An adjective, referring to herbs, as in an herbal tea.

   2. A noun, usually reflecting the botanical or medicinal aspects of herbs; also a book which catalogs and illustrates herbs.

   The word "herbal" was pronounced with a silent h on both sides of the Atlantic until the nineteenth century, but this usage persists only on the American side.

407)   **High blood pressure:** Also known as hypertension, high blood pressure is, by definition, a repeatedly elevated blood pressure exceeding 140 over 90 mmHg—a systolic pressure above 140 with a diastolic pressure above 90.

408)   **Hormone:** A chemical substance produced in the body that controls and regulates the activity of certain cells or organs.

409)   **Hypercholesterolemia:** High blood cholesterol. This can be sporadic (with no family history) or familial.

410)   **Hypertension:** High blood pressure, defined as a repeatedly elevated blood pressure exceeding 140 over 90 mmHg—a systolic pressure above 140 with a diastolic pressure above 90.

411)   **Hypothyroid:** Deficiency of thyroid hormone which is normally made by the thyroid gland which is located in the front of the neck.

412) **Incidence:** The frequency with which something, such as a disease, appears in a particular population or area. In disease epidemiology, the incidence is the number of newly diagnosed cases during a specific time period. The incidence is distinct from the *prevalence* which refers to the number of cases alive on a certain date.

413) **Infection:** The growth of a parasitic organism within the body. (A parasitic organism is one that lives on or in another organism and draws its nourishment therefrom.) A person with an infection has another organism (a "germ") growing within him, drawing its nourishment from the person.

414) *http://www.medicinenet.com/obesity_weight_loss/glossary.htm–backtotop* Injury: Harm or hurt. The term "injury" may be applied in medicine to damage inflicted upon oneself as in a *hamstring injury* or by an external agent on as in a *cold injury*. The injury may be accidental or deliberate, as with a *needlestick injury*. The term "injury" may be synonymous (depending on the context) with a wound or with *trauma*.

415) **Insomnia:** The perception or complaint of inadequate or poor-quality sleep because of one or more of the following: difficulty falling asleep; waking up frequently during the night with difficulty returning to sleep; waking up too early in the morning; or unrefreshing sleep. Insomnia is not defined by the number of hours of sleep a person gets or how long it takes to fall asleep. Individuals vary normally in their need for, and their satisfaction with, sleep. Insomnia may cause problems during the day, such as tiredness, a lack of energy, difficulty concentrating, and irritability.

416) **Insulin:** A natural hormone made by the pancreas that controls the level of the sugar glucose in the blood. Insulin permits cells to use glucose for energy. Cells cannot utilize glucose without insulin.

417) **Insulin resistance:** The diminished ability of cells to respond to the action of *insulin* in transporting *glucose* (sugar) from the bloodstream into *muscle* and other tissues. Insulin resistance typically develops with *obesity* and heralds the onset of *type 2*

diabetes. It is as if insulin is "knocking" on the door of muscle. The muscle hears the knock, opens up, and lets glucose in. But with insulin resistance, the muscle cannot hear the knocking of the insulin (the muscle is "resistant"). The *pancreas* makes more insulin which increases insulin levels in the blood and causes a louder "knock." Eventually, the pancreas produces far more insulin than normal, and the muscles continue to be resistant to the knock. As long as one can produce enough insulin to overcome this resistance, blood glucose levels remain normal. Once the pancreas is no longer able to keep up, blood glucose starts to rise, initially after meals, eventually even in the fasting state. Type 2 diabetes is now overt.

418) **Iron:** An essential mineral. Iron is necessary for the transport of oxygen (via hemoglobin in red blood cells) and for oxidation by cells (via cytochrome). Deficiency of iron is a common cause of *anemia.* Food sources of iron include meat, poultry, eggs, vegetables, and cereals (especially those fortified with iron). According to the National Academy of Sciences, the recommended dietary allowances of iron are 15 milligrams per day for women and 10 milligrams per day for men. Iron overload can damage the heart, liver, gonads, and other organs. Iron overload is a particular risk in people who may have certain genetic conditions (*hemochromatosis*) sometimes without knowing it and also in people receiving recurrent blood transfusions. Iron supplements meant for adults (such as pregnant women) are a major cause of poisoning in children.

419) **Large bowel:** Another name for the large intestine.

420) **Lean body mass:** The mass of the body minus the fat (storage *lipid*). There are a number of methods for determining the lean body mass. Some of these methods require specialized equipment such as underwater weighing (hydrostatic weighing), BOD POD (a computerized chamber), and DEXA (dual-energy x-ray absorptiometry). Other methods for determining the lean body mass are simple such as skin calipers and bioelectric impedance analysis (BIA).

421) **Leptin:** A hormone that has a central role in fat metabolism. Leptin was originally thought to be a signal to lose weight, but it may, instead, be a signal to the brain that there is fat on the body.

422) **Lumen:** A luminous term referring to the channel within a tube such as a blood vessel or to the cavity within a hollow organ such as the intestine. Lumen is a luminous term because it is Latin for light, including the light that comes through a window. When a hollow organ is cut across, you can see light through the space that has been opened. So the word "lumen" came to mean this space.

423) **Lungs:** The lungs are a pair of breathing organs located with the chest which remove carbon dioxide from and bring oxygen to the blood. There is a right and left lung.

424) **Malnutrition:** A term used to refer to any condition in which the body does not receive enough nutrients for proper function. Malnutrition may range from mild to severe and life-threatening. It can be a result of starvation in which a person has an inadequate intake of calories, or it may be related to a deficiency of one particular nutrient (for example, vitamin C deficiency). Malnutrition can also occur because a person cannot properly digest or absorb nutrients from the food they consume, as may occur with certain medical conditions. Malnutrition remains a significant global problem, especially in developing countries.

425) **Marker:** A piece of DNA that lies on a chromosome so close to a gene that the marker and the gene are inherited together. A marker is thus an identifiable heritable spot on a chromosome. A marker can be an expressed region of DNA (a gene) or a segment of DNA with no known coding function. All that matters is that the marker can be detected and trailed.

426) **Menopause:** The time in a woman's life when menstrual periods permanently stop; it is also called the "change of life." Menopause is the opposite of the menarche.

427) **Menstrual cycle:** The monthly cycle of changes in the ovaries and the lining of the uterus (endometrium), starting with the preparation of an egg for fertilization. When the follicle of the prepared egg in the ovary breaks, it is released for fertilization and ovulation occurs. Unless pregnancy occurs, the cycle ends with the shedding of part of the endometrium, which is menstruation. Although it is actually the end of the physical cycle, the first day of menstrual bleeding is designated as "day 1" of the menstrual cycle in medical parlance.

428) *http://www.medicinenet.com/obesity_weight_loss/glossary.htm–backtotop*
Metabolic: Relating to metabolism, the whole range of biochemical processes that occur within us (or any living organism). Metabolism consists of anabolism (the buildup of substances) and catabolism (the breakdown of substances).

429) **Metabolism:** The whole range of biochemical processes that occur within us (or any living organism). Metabolism consists both of anabolism and catabolism (the buildup and breakdown of substances, respectively). The term is commonly used to refer specifically to the breakdown of food and its transformation into energy.

430) **Mortality:** A fatal outcome or, in one word, death. The word "mortality" is derived from "mortal" which came from the Latin word, *mors* (death). The opposite of mortality is, of course, immortality. Mortality is also quite distinct from morbidity (illness).

431) **Muscle:** Muscle is the tissue of the body which primarily functions as a source of power. There are three types of muscle in the body. Muscle which is responsible for moving extremities and external areas of the body is called skeletal muscle. Heart muscle is called cardiac muscle. Muscle that is in the walls of arteries and bowel is called smooth muscle.

432) **Muscular:** Having to do with the muscles. Also, endowed with above-average muscle development. Muscular system refers to all of the muscles of the body collectively.

433)   **Nerve:** A bundle of fibers that uses chemical and electrical signals to transmit sensory and motor information from one body part to another. See *Nervous system*.

434)   **Normal range:** By convention, the normal range for whatever (a particular test, condition, symptom, behavior, etc.) is set to cover 95 percent of all values from the general population. Five percent of results consequently fall outside the normal range. Values that prove normal can therefore sometimes be outside the normal range.

435)   **Nurses Health Study:** A very large and important prospective investigation into the risk factors for major chronic diseases in women. (In a prospective study, the participants are identified and then followed forward in time.) The participants in the study are female registered nurses (RNs).

436   **Nutrition:** 1) The science or practice of taking in and utilizing foods. 2) A nourishing substance, such as nutritional solutions delivered to hospitalized patients via an IV or IG tube.

437)   **Obese:** Well above one's normal weight. A person has traditionally been considered to be obese if they are more than 20 percent over their ideal weight. That ideal weight must take into account the person's height, age, sex, and build.

438)   **Obesity:** The state of being well above one's normal weight.

439)   **Onset:** In medicine, the first appearance of the signs or symptoms of an illness as, for example, the onset of rheumatoid arthritis. There is always an onset to a disease but never to the return to good health. The default setting is good health.

440)   **Organ:** A relatively independent part of the body that carries out one or more special functions. The organs of the human body include the *eye, ear, heart, lungs,* and *liver*.

441)   **Osteoarthritis:** A type of arthritis caused by inflammation, breakdown, and eventual loss of cartilage in the joints. Also known as degenerative arthritis.

442) **Osteoporosis:** Thinning of the bones with reduction in bone mass due to depletion of calcium and bone protein. Osteoporosis predisposes a person to fractures which are often slow to heal and heal poorly. It is more common in older adults, particularly postmenopausal women, in patients on steroids, and in those who take steroidal drugs. Unchecked osteoporosis can lead to changes in posture, physical abnormality (particularly the form of hunched back known colloquially as "dowager's hump"), and decreased mobility.

443) *http://www.medicinenet.com/obesity_weight_loss/glossary.htm–backtotop*
Ovary: The female gonad, the ovary is one of a pair of reproductive glands in women. They are located in the pelvis, one on each side of the uterus. Each ovary is about the size and shape of an almond. The ovaries produce eggs (ova) and female hormones. During each monthly menstrual cycle, an egg is released from one ovary. The egg travels from the ovary through a fallopian tube to the uterus. The ovaries are the main source of female hormones which control the development of female body characteristics, such as the breasts, body shape, and body hair. They also regulate the menstrual cycle and pregnancy.

444) **Overweight:** The term "overweight" is used in two different ways. In one sense, it is a way of saying imprecisely that someone is heavy. The other sense of "overweight" is more precise and designates a state between normal weight and obesity.

445) **Pain:** An unpleasant sensation that can range from mild, localized discomfort to agony. Pain has both physical and emotional components. The physical part of pain results from nerve stimulation. Pain may be contained to a discrete area, as in an injury, or it can be more diffuse, as in disorders like fibromyalgia. Pain is mediated by specific nerve fibers that carry the pain impulses to the brain where their conscious appreciation may be modified by many factors.

446) **Pancreas:** A fish-shaped spongy grayish-pink organ about 6 inches (15 cm) long that stretches across the back of the abdomen, behind the stomach. The head of the pancreas is on the right side of the abdomen and is connected to the duodenum (the first section of the small intestine). The narrow end of the pancreas, called the tail, extends to the left side of the body.

447) **Phenylalanine:** An essential amino acid. (The human body cannot make it, so it is essential to the diet.) Phenylalanine that is ingested is largely transformed (hydroxylated) to form the amino acid tyrosine which is used in protein synthesis. Too little phenylalanine curbs physical and intellectual growth. Too much phenylalanine, as in phenylketonuria (PKU), is highly toxic to the brain. Phenylanine was first isolated in 1879 and first synthesized in 1882. Symbol: Phe.

448) **Phenylketonuria:** The inherited inability to metabolize (process) the essential amino acid phenylalanine due to complete or near-complete deficiency of the enzyme phenylalanine hydroxylase.

449) **Placenta:** A temporary organ joining the mother and fetus, the placenta transfers oxygen and nutrients from the mother to the fetus and permits the release of carbon dioxide and waste products from the fetus. It is roughly disk-shaped, and at full term measures about seven inches in diameter and a bit less than two inches thick. The upper surface of the placenta is smooth, while the under surface is rough. The placenta is rich in blood vessels.

450) **Polycystic Ovary Syndrome:** Abbreviated as PCOS. Polcystic ovary syndrome is a condition in women characterized by irregular or no menstrual periods, acne, obesity, and excess hair growth. PCOS is a disorder of chronically abnormal ovarian function and hyperandrogenism (abnormally elevated androgen levels). It affects 5 to 10 percent of women of reproductive age. PCOS is also called the Stein-Leventhal syndrome.

451) **Postmenopausal:** After the menopause. Postmenopausal is defined formally as the time after which a woman has experienced twelve (12) consecutive months of amenorrhea (lack of menstruation) without a period.

452) **Potassium:** The major positive ion (cation) found inside of cells. The chemical notation for potassium is K^+.

453) **Pound:** A measure of weight equal to 16 ounces or, metrically, 453.6 grams. The word "pound" goes back to the Latin *pondo* which meant a "weight" (but one of only 12 ounces). The abbreviation for pound—just to confuse nonpound people—is *lb.* which stands for "libra" (Latin for pound).

454) **Pregnancy:** The state of carrying a developing embryo or fetus within the female body. This condition can be indicated by positive results on an over-the-counter urine test and confirmed through a blood test, ultrasound, detection of fetal heartbeat, or an x-ray. Pregnancy lasts for about nine months, measured from the date of the woman's last menstrual period (LMP). It is conventionally divided into three trimesters, each roughly three months long.

455) **Pregnant:** The state of carrying a developing fetus within the body.

456) **Prescription:** A physician's order for the preparation and administration of a drug or device for a patient. A prescription has several parts. They include the superscription or heading with the symbol *R* or *Rx*, which stands for the word recipe (meaning, in Latin, to take); the inscription, which contains the names and quantities of the ingredients; the subscription or directions for compounding the drug; and the signature which is often preceded by the sign *s* standing for signa (Latin for mark), giving the directions to be marked on the container.

457) **Prevalence:** The proportion of individuals in a population having a disease. Prevalence is a statistical concept referring to the number of cases of a disease that are present in a particular population at a given time.

458)   *http://www.medicinenet.com/obesity_weight_loss/glossary.htm–backtotop*
Prospective: Looking forward. A prospective study or a prospective clinical trial is one in which the participants are identified and then followed forward in time.

459)   **Prospective study:** A study in which the subjects are identified and then followed forward in time.

460)   **Prostate:** A gland within the male reproductive system that is located just below the bladder. Chestnut-shaped, the prostate surrounds the beginning of the urethra, the canal that empties the bladder.

461)   **Protein:** A large molecule composed of one or more chains of amino acids in a specific order determined by the base sequence of nucleotides in the DNA coding for the protein.

462)   **Pulmonary:** Having to do with the lungs. (The word comes from the Latin *pulmo* for lung.)

463)   **Pulmonary hypertension:** High blood pressure in the pulmonary artery that conveys blood from the right ventricle to the lungs. The pressure in the pulmonary artery is normally low compared to that in the aorta. Pulmonary hypertension can irrevocably damage the lungs and cause failure of the right ventricle.

464)   **Rectum:** The last 6 to 8 inches of the large intestine. The rectum stores solid waste until it leaves the body through the anus. The word rectum comes from the Latin *rectus* meaning straight (which the human rectum is not).

465)   **Regimen:** With the accent on the first syllable (reg as in Reggie Jackson), a regimen is a plan, a regulated course such as a diet, exercise or treatment, designed to give a good result. A low-salt diet is a regimen.

466)   **Relapse:** The return of signs and symptoms of a disease after a patient has enjoyed a remission. For example, after treatment, a patient with cancer of the colon went into remission with no sign or symptom of the tumor, remained in remission for four years but then suffered a relapse and had to be treated once again for colon cancer.

467) **Resistance:** Opposition to something or the ability to withstand it. For example, some forms of staphylococcus are resistant to treatment with antibiotics.

468) **Saccharin:** An artificial sweetener which diluted in water is three hundred to five hundred times sweeter than the sugar sucrose. (The chemical name for saccharin is o-sulfabenzamide; 2, 3-dihydro-3-oxobenzisosulfonazole).

469) **Saturated fat:** A fat that is solid at room temperature and comes chiefly from animal food products. Some examples are butter, lard, meat fat, solid shortening, palm oil, and coconut oil. These fats tend to raise the level of cholesterol in the blood.

470) **Sensation:** In medicine and physiology, sensation refers to the registration of an incoming (afferent) nerve impulse in that part of the brain called the sensorium which is capable of such perception. Therefore, the awareness of a stimulus as a result of its perception by sensory receptors. (Sensory here is synonymous with sensation.)

471) **Sensitivity: 1.** In psychology, the quality of being sensitive. As, for example, sensitivity training, training in small groups to develop a sensitive awareness and understanding of oneself and of one's relationships with others. **2.** In disease epidemiology, the ability of a system to detect epidemics and other changes in disease occurrence. **3.** In screening for a disease, the proportion of persons with the disease who are correctly identified by a screening test. **4.** In the definition of a disease, the proportion of persons with the disease who are correctly identified by defined criteria.

472) *http://www.medicinenet.com/obesity_weight_loss/glossary.htm—backtotop* **Serotonin:** A hormone, also called 5-hydroxytryptamine, in the pineal gland, blood platelets, the digestive tract, and the brain. Serotonin acts both as a chemical messenger that transmits nerve signals between nerve cells and that causes blood vessels to narrow.

473) **Shock:** In medicine, shock is a critical condition brought on by a sudden drop in blood flow through the body. There

is failure of the circulatory system to maintain adequate blood flow. This sharply curtails the delivery of oxygen and nutrients to vital organs. It also compromises the kidney and so curtails the removal of wastes from the body. Shock can be due to a number of different mechanisms including not enough blood volume (hypovolemic shock) and not enough output of blood by the heart (cardiogenic shock). The signs and symptoms of shock include low blood pressure (hypotension), overbreathing (hyperventilation), a weak rapid pulse, cold clammy grayish-bluish (cyanotic) skin, decreased urine flow (oliguria), and mental changes (a sense of great anxiety and foreboding, confusion and, sometimes, combativeness).

474) **Shortness of breath:** Difficulty in breathing. Medically, it is referred to as *dyspnea*. Shortness of breath can be caused by respiratory (breathing passages and lungs) or circulatory (heartand blood vessels) conditions.

475) **Skin calipers:** A simple method for determining the lean body mass. This method involves measuring the skinfold thickness of the layer of fat just under the skin in several parts of the body with calipers. The results are then calculated, and the percentage of body fat is determined. Skin calipers can yield inaccurate results if an inexperienced person uses them on someone with significant obesity.

476) **Sleep:** The body's rest cycle.

477) **Sleep apnea:** The temporary stoppage of breathing during sleep, often resulting in daytime sleepiness. Apnea is a Greek word that means "want of breath."

478) **Small bowel:** Another name for the small intestine.

479) **Sodium:** The major positive ion (cation) in fluid outside of cells. The chemical notation for sodium is Na^+. When combined with chloride, the resulting substance is table salt.

480) **Stomach:** 1. The sac-shaped digestive organ that is located in the upper abdomen under the ribs. The upper part of the stomach connects to the esophagus, and the lower part leads into the small intestine.

481) **Stress:** Forces from the outside world impinging on the individual. Stress is a normal part of life that can help us learn and grow. Conversely, stress can cause us significant problems.

482) **Stroke:** The sudden death of some brain cells due to a lack of oxygen when the blood flow to the brain is impaired by blockage or rupture of an artery to the brain. A stroke is also called a cerebrovascular accident or, for short, a CVA.

483) **Surgery:** The word "surgery" has multiple meanings. It is the branch of medicine concerned with diseases and conditions which require or are amenable to operative procedures. Surgery is the work done by a surgeon. By analogy, the work of an editor wielding his pen as a scalpel is s form of surgery. A surgery in England (and some other countries) is a physician's or dentist's office.

484) **Sympathetic nervous system:** A part of the nervous system that serves to accelerate the heart rate, constrict blood vessels, and raise blood pressure. The sympathetic nervous system and the parasympathetic nervous system constitute the autonomic nervous system, the branch of the nervous system that performs involuntary functions.

485) **Synapse:** The point of connection usually between two nerve cells. Specifically, a synapse is a specialized junction at which a nerve cell (a neuron) communicates with a target cell. The neuron releases a chemical transmitter (a neurotransmitter) that diffuses across a small gap and activates specific specialized sites called receptors situated on the target cell. The target cell may be another neuron or a specialized region of a muscle cell or a secretory cell (a cell that can make and secrete a substance). Neurons can also communicate through direct electrical connections (electrical synapses).

486) **Syndrome:** A set of signs and symptoms that tend to occur together and which reflect the presence of a particular disease or an increased chance of developing a particular disease.

487) *http://www.medicinenet.com/obesity_weight_loss/glossary.htm–backtotop*
Systemic: Affecting the entire body. A systemic disease such as diabetes can affect the whole body.

Systemic *chemotherapy* employs drugs that travel through the bloodstream and reach and affect cells all over the body.

488) **Thrombosis:** The formation or presence of a *blood clot* in blood *vessel*. The vessel may be any *vein* or *artery* as, for example, in a deep vein thrombosis or a coronary (artery) thrombosis. The clot itself is termed a *thrombus*. If the clot breaks loose and travels through the bloodstream, it is a thromboembolism. Thrombosis, *thrombus*, and the prefix *thrombo* all come from the Greek *thrombos*, meaning a lump or clump, or a curd or clot of milk. See entries also *Cavernous sinus thrombosis; Renal vein thrombosis.*

489) **Thyroid: 1.** The thyroid gland. Also pertaining to the thyroid gland. **2.** A preparation of the thyroid gland used to treat hypothyroidism. **3.** Shaped like a shield. (The thyroid gland was so named by Thomas Wharton in 1656 because it was shaped like an ancient Greek shield.)

490) **Transplant:** The grafting of a tissue from one place to another, just as in botany, a bud from one plant might be grafted onto the stem of another. The transplanting of tissue can be from one part of the patient to another (autologous transplantation), as in the case of a skin graft using the patient's own skin, or from one patient to another (allogenic transplantation), as in the case of transplanting a donor kidney into a recipient.

491) **Treadmill:** A machine with a moving strip on which one walks without moving forward. A treadmill was originally a wide wheel turned by the weight of people climbing on steps around its edge, used in the past to provide power for machines or as a punishment in prisons.

492) **Underwater weighing:** A method for determining the *lean body mass*. This method weighs a person underwater and then calculates the lean body mass (muscle) and body fat. This method is one of the more accurate ones. However, it is generally done in special research facilities, and the equipment is costly. Also called hydrostatic weighing.

493) **Uterus:** The uterus (womb) is a hollow, pear-shaped organ located in a woman's lower abdomen between the bladder

and the rectum. The narrow lower portion of the uterus is the cervix; the broader upper part is the corpus. The corpus is made up of two layers of tissue.

494) **Vein:** A blood vessel that carries blood low in oxygen content from the body back to the heart. The deoxygenated form of hemoglobin (deoxyhemoglobin) in venous blood makes it appear dark. Veins are part of the afferent wing of the circulatory system which returns blood to the heart.

495) **Vitamins:** The word "vitamin" was coined in 1911 by the Warsaw-born biochemist Casimir Funk (1884–1967). At the Lister Institute in London, Funk isolated a substance that prevented nerve inflammation (neuritis) in chickens raised on a diet deficient in that substance. He named the substance *vitamine* because he believed it was necessary to life, and it was a chemical amine. The *e* at the end was later removed when it was recognized that vitamins need not be amines.

496) **Weight loss:** Weight loss is a decrease in body weight resulting from either voluntary (diet, exercise) or involuntary (illness) circumstances. Most instances of *weight loss* arise due to the loss of body fat, but in cases of extreme or severe weight loss, protein and other substances in the body can also be depleted. Examples of involuntary weight loss include the weight loss associated with *cancer*, *malabsorption* (such as from chronic diarrhea), and chronic *inflammation* (such as with rheumatoid arthritis).

497) **World Health Organization:** An agency of the United Nations established in 1948 to further international cooperation in improving health conditions. Although the World Health Organization inherited specific tasks relating to epidemic control, quarantine measures, and drug standardization from the Health Organization of the League of Nations (that was set up in 1923) and from the International Office of Public Health at Paris (established in 1909), the World Health Organization was given a broad mandate under its constitution to promote the attainment of "the highest possible level of health" by all people. WHO

defines health positively as "a state of complete physical, mental, and social well-being and not merely the absence of disease or infirmity."

498) **Wrist:** The proximal segment (the near part) of the hand consisting of the carpal bones and the associated soft parts.

499) **X-ray: 1.** High-energy radiation with waves shorter than those of visible light. X-rays possess the properties of penetrating most substances (to varying extents), of acting on a photographic film or plate (permitting radiography), and of causing a fluorescent screen to give off light (permitting fluoroscopy). In low doses, x-rays are used for making images that help to diagnose disease, and in high doses to treat cancer. Formerly called a Roentgen ray. **2.** An image obtained by means of x-rays.

500) **Xylitol:** A sweetener found in plants that is used as a substitute for sugar. Xylitol is considered a nutritive sweetener because it provides calories, just like sugar. (*Saccharin* is an example of a nonnutritive sweetener, one that has no calories.)

Other Interesting Facts

501) Four foods that you should never eat: sugar, whole wheat, margarine, and processed foods.

502) Alabama wants to tax fat people.

503) Women tend to gain weight faster than men after a diet.

504) For fat women, 95 percent is impossible to say no for lack of self-esteem.

505) People gain weight almost immediately after marriage.

506) There are more of a hundred reasons known to accumulate weight.

507) Obesity, besides the usual illnesses, also develops genetic deviations and a lot of hormonal disorders.

508) Stress causes obesity.

509)   In France, 40 percent of the people from fourteen years old to twenty years old do not accept the way they look thanks to obesity.

510)   There is a large movement to tax fat people that have at least 30 or more BMI.

511)   Against common knowledge, chubby and fat people are not "jolly."

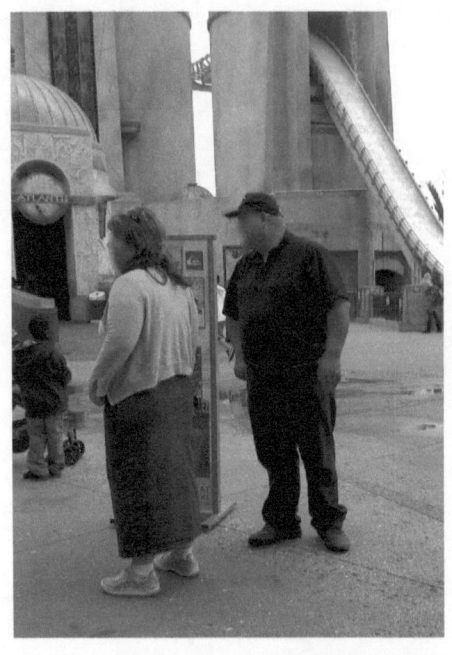

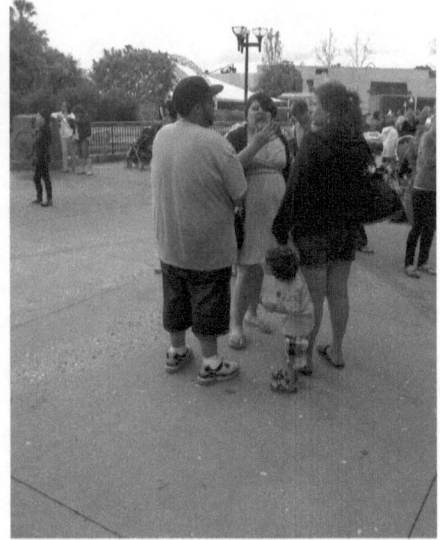

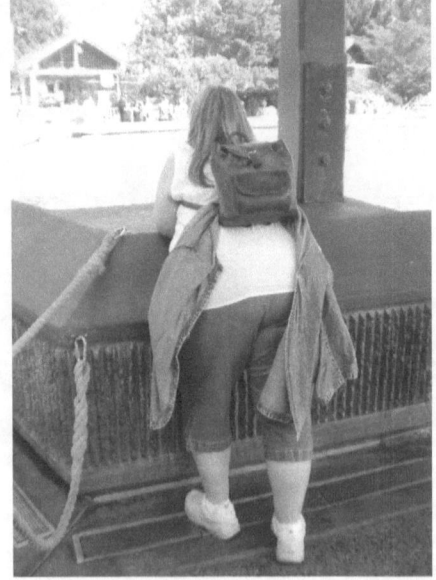

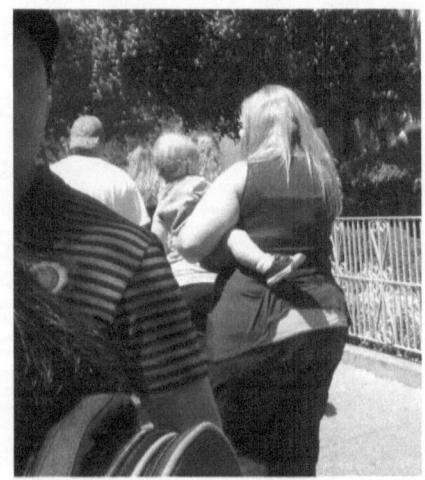

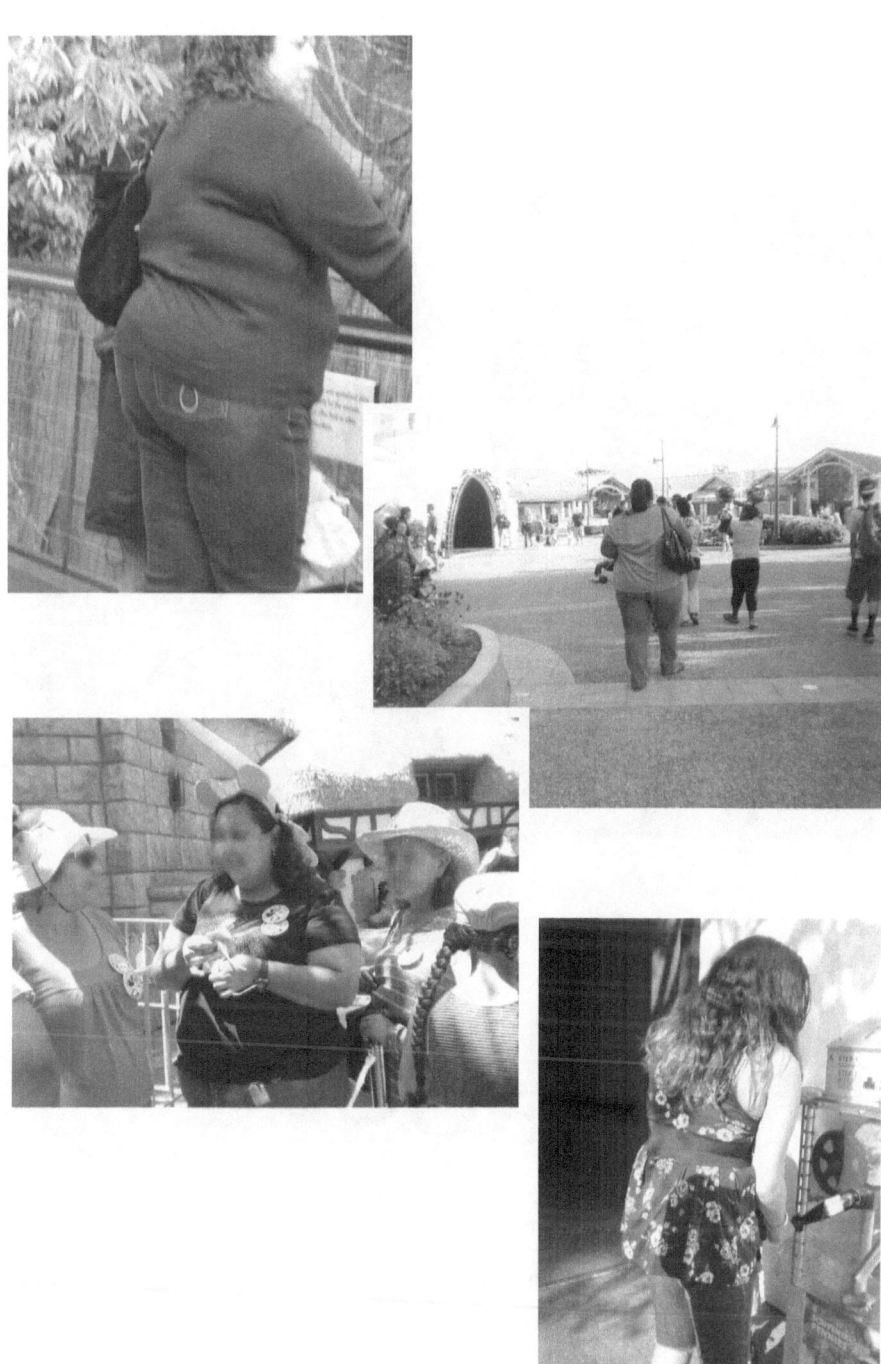

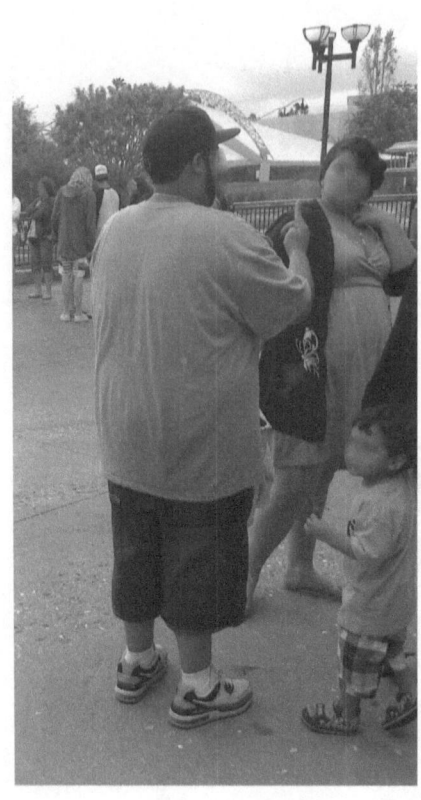 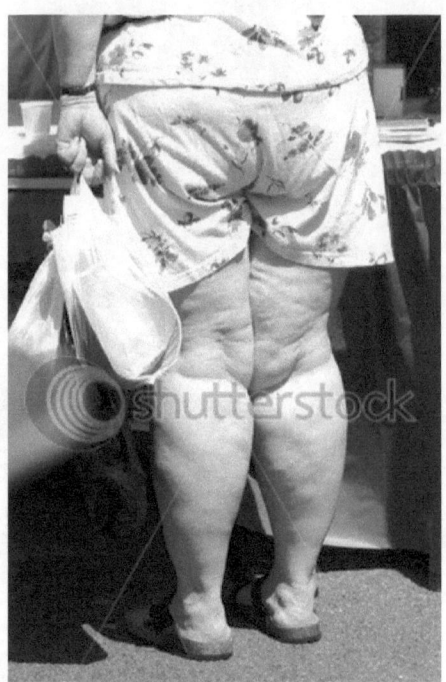

www.ingramcontent.com/pod-product-compliance
Lightning Source LLC
Chambersburg PA
CBHW031255280526
45784CB00004B/1860